REIMAGINED MOTHERHOOD

UNTRIGGERED

FARRAH FAYE

Disclaimer

This book is intended for informational purposes only and is not a substitute for professional advice, diagnosis, or treatment in any field, including medical, psychological, legal, or financial areas. Exercise, dietary, and product suggestions should be tailored to individual circumstances, and readers should consult qualified professionals before making changes. This book is not a replacement for therapy or other mental health services.

The information reflects knowledge at the time of publication. The author and publisher are not responsible for changes, inaccuracies, or the availability of referenced resources. Mention of entities, trademarks, or organizations does not imply endorsement or affiliation.

The author and publisher disclaim all liability for any actions taken based on this book. Results may vary, and readers accept full responsibility for their own well-being and actions.

No part of this book may be reproduced, stored in a retrieval system, or transmitted in any form or by any means, electronic, mechanical, photocopying, recording, or otherwise, without prior written permission from the publisher, except for brief quotations used in reviews or permitted under copyright law.

REIMAGINED MOTHERHOOD: UNTRIGGERED.

Copyright © 2024 The Pivot North Publishing. All rights reserved.
ISBN 979-8-9920794-0-1
Library of Congress Control Number: 2024925233

Access your printable resources and other freebies by scanning this QR code:

DEDICATION

You — the one still searching.
You — the inner child who longs to be seen and heard.
You — the one who has braved so much in this life.

This is for you.

Table of Contents

Introduction 1

Chapter X – The Apology Unspoken 5

Chapter 1 – To Understand Your 'SELF', Start Here 13

Chapter 2 – The Invisible Load of Motherhood 23

Chapter 3 – The Baggage I Didn't Know I Had 37

Chapter 4 – The Invisible Saboteurs 83

Chapter 5 – You're Not Okay 95

Chapter 6 – Your Brain Isn't Your Bestie 109

Chapter 7 – Life Happens for You 133

Chapter 8 – Self-Care Unplugged: Am I Being True to Myself? 147

Chapter 9 – Calm Blueprint 159

Chapter 10 – Creating a Supportive Environment 163

Chapter 11 – Setting Boundaries with Love 173

Chapter 12 – Embracing and Transforming Shame, Guilt, and Anger 185

Chapter 13 – Embracing Self-Compassion 199

Chapter 14 – The Weight of Your Own Story 211

Chapter 15 – Tools for Healing: Practical Techniques for Transformation . 219

Conclusion – A Heartfelt Thank You 251

References 255

Acknowledgements 271

Introduction

Spend a moment gently closing your eyes and taking a deep breath, letting yourself fully relax. Imagine a warm, comforting presence beside you, like reconnecting with an old friend after a long time apart, picking up right where you left off. Life can be overwhelming with its constant demand and I get it. It's easy to feel stressed and disconnected. But by opening this book, you've already made a courageous choice to find some peace and make your journey a little easier.

Settle in your cozy spot where you can truly unwind. Treat yourself to a warm, soothing drink and wrap yourself in a soft, comforting blanket. Let's sit together and have a heartfelt conversation about gently lightening your responsibilities, embracing your unique qualities, and truly honoring the amazing mother you are.

By the time you complete this book, I will have been a mother for 7,590 days. And that doesn't even include the years I spent caring for my siblings before having my own children. I was just 22 when I experienced the most incredible bliss of my life. I was blessed with four more wonderful gifts, and my journey since then has been unimaginable. It's been a path filled with moments of pure joy and invaluable lessons that I will carry with me forever. Admittedly, I've equally faced challenges that taught me hard truths.

Looking back, I realize there were parts of me that needed nurturing, guidance, and understanding that I didn't even know I was missing.

This book isn't about offering a flawless manual or a one-size-fits-all solution. It's not about trying to reach some impossible standard. Instead, it's a gentle reminder to help you navigate the challenges of motherhood with a bit more ease and insight. If you've already made some of the mistakes I discuss, please know that you're not alone. We've all had moments where we wish we could have done things differently. I certainly do. It's hard not to feel sad when I think about how much easier and calmer my early years of parenting could have been if I had someone to offer me guidance. But it's never too late to make a positive change. With a heart full of love and a deep concern for mothers like you, who would sacrifice anything for their children, this book is here to provide the support and encouragement you need, no matter where you are on your journey.

Remember, my friend, that your well-being is at the heart of this book. You are truly cherished and appreciated in these pages. If, at any point, you find yourself confronting heavy feelings you've held onto for a long time, know it's perfectly okay to release and let go. You're in a supportive environment where you can freely explore your emotions and discover ways to heal.

Perhaps your children are grown now, maybe even starting families of their own. No matter where you are in your journey, the insights and strategies in this book can still help. They can guide you in strengthening your relationships with your adult children and their families. It's never too late to deepen those connections, look out for their well-being, or come to peace with the decisions you've made in the past.

Every step you take toward understanding and healing is a step toward a more fulfilling and empowered life. My faith has been a steady source of strength through all the highs and lows of life, of motherhood. I hope these pages bring you the wisdom and encouragement to parent confidently, raise happy, resilient children, and find your own peace along the way.

If you are in the storm right now, I encourage you to seek comfort and strength in what brings you peace. For me, that has meant throwing myself into God's loving arms. He has been my anchor, my refuge, and my strength. Together, we'll face the tough aspects of motherhood. Together we'll confront past challenges, and explore practical ways to bring calm and joy into your daily life. I've included personal stories and insights gathered over the years, alongside scientifically backed research, to support the concepts written here. This book serves as your personal guide to a lighter, more graceful journey.

You'll notice certain concepts, ideas, or phrases being repeated. This is intentional and done with care. Real change happens when important messages are revisited and allowed to take root in your heart and mind. By consistently reflecting on these concepts, you'll create a foundation that supports your growth in a way that feels natural and lasting. It's about making gentle progress, not about being perfect.

So, take a moment to celebrate every little win, even if it's just getting through the day with a smile. I'll always be here to remind you to appreciate each step you take forward. Be kind to yourself, and when you look in the mirror, give yourself a little high five—you've earned it. Your commitment to personal growth and your dedication to making a positive difference show just how strong and resilient you truly are.

Are you ready to go on this journey? You are empowered to make significant changes, and I'll be here to support you every step of the way.

CHAPTER X

The Apology Unspoken

A Glimpse into the Past

As a child, I watched with a knot in my stomach as other children ran into their parents' arms—moms and dads who brought them lunch, picked them up from school, and cheered them on at school events. But instead of feeling the good kind of butterflies, my stomach churned with a painful flutter. Those moments—reciting poems, singing songs, dancing in plays—were when I wanted to feel seen. I wanted to feel important too, like the other kids. Every passing year during these events, I found myself standing alone, looking through the crowd of faces for someone who would never arrive.

It was in these early years that the seeds of envy and loneliness were planted within me. But these were not the only seeds sown in the quiet spaces of my heart. Alongside them came roots of deep self-doubt and a lingering feeling of unworthiness, subtly entangled with my lack of sense of self. I didn't understand why I felt such a deep ache when I saw the other children surrounded by love. All I knew was that their joy highlighted the emptiness I felt. I became used to masking my pain, pretending it didn't matter, but deep down, the wounds festered. As I grew older, that envy and loneliness took shape in ways I couldn't recognize at the time. I would see others' happiness, their close relationships, their successes, and feel a pang of something I could not quite name—a mixture of longing, resentment, and sadness.

Running Away: A Cry for Safety

In my desperate attempts to escape these overwhelming feelings, I ran away from home several times during my childhood. Each time, I hoped to find somewhere, anywhere, that felt safer, more secure, and more loving than the place I was fleeing from. My home, which should have been a sanctuary, felt anything but safe due to a violation that shattered my sense of security. The fear and anxiety I felt upon being sent back home was crippling. The thought alone of being in the same environment was terrifying and chilling to the bone. The thought of getting into trouble for running away seemed trivial compared to the turmoil that would torment my mind when I was forced back into that house. It wasn't just a cry for attention; it was a desperate attempt to escape the mental and emotional turmoil I was enduring and to find even a fleeting sense of safety and belonging.

This pattern of running away didn't end with my childhood. Throughout my teens and even into adulthood, I found myself retreating from situations that felt overwhelming. Whether it was emotionally charged arguments, challenging relationships, or moments of intense self-reflection, my instinct was to escape—to hide from the feelings and emotions that surfaced. It wasn't until much later in adulthood that I came to realize I needed to confront these deeply ingrained issues. The cycle of avoidance was both frustrating and familiar; I was evading the very problems I needed to address. Running away became a well-worn defense mechanism, a shield to protect me from the pain I wasn't yet ready to face.

The Unspoken Apology

Now, as I reflect on those years and the person I became, I realize that my unresolved pain from childhood didn't just fade away—it followed me like a shadow, impacting every aspect of my life. The influence of those early experiences molded my perspective and, more deeply, affected how I related to others.

Early years of frequent betrayal and mistreatment left me with a profound feeling of abandonment that colored everything I saw and felt. I lived in a state of constant fear and unease, as if every interaction might bring more pain. When I pulled away or acted out, it wasn't just about the moment at hand; it was a reflection of the wounds I carried with me. I felt distant, not because I didn't care but because my own pain and insecurities were so overwhelming that it made it hard to connect. I felt like I was constantly bracing for more hurt, as if showing any softness would just open me up to more rejection. No way I was going to allow that. The unpleasantness you saw from me was my way of trying to protect myself from feeling even more vulnerable. Inside, there was a desperate yearning to be truly seen and heard, but I was trapped in a cycle of self-protection and isolation, longing for the connection and acceptance that always seemed just out of reach.

And when I found myself envying others instead of celebrating them, it was a reflection of the internal struggle I faced. It wasn't about you—it was about the emptiness I felt inside. This inner battle made it challenging for me to embrace others' joy while dealing with my own feelings of disconnection. My inability to genuinely rejoice in your successes or share in your happiness was a direct result of the unresolved feelings of inadequacy and sorrow that I hadn't yet dealt with.

I deeply regret the times when my actions or attitudes may have hurt others. My behavior was often a misguided attempt to protect myself or cope with emotions I didn't fully understand. It wasn't a true reflection of our relationship. I now realize that the pain I tried so hard to hide or outrun inadvertently affected those around me. For the times I fell short of being my best self and couldn't offer you the support or kindness you deserved I sincerely apologize.

This apology is not about making excuses but about shedding light on the struggles I faced. It wasn't just the adult me dealing with others; it was also the wounded inner child within me. The child who felt unseen, unworthy, and unsafe—longing for affection, acceptance, and protection but often met with silence or rejection. I wanted to connect more closely at times, but I found myself pulling away because I was carrying the weight of silent fears. I found it difficult to welcome the joy in other people's lives because I felt so cut off from myself.

To the friends who felt the sting of my distance, the loved ones who endured my harshness, and those who sensed my envy and jealousy when they deserved my support I offer this apology. Please know this is not an excuse but an explanation. I was doing the best I knew how, navigating a world that seemed to offer everyone else what felt beyond my grasp.

A Shared Experience

I'm sharing this because I believe that many of us carry these hidden pains—wounds from the past that manifest in ways we may not even recognize. We try to move forward, to build our lives and relationships, but those old feelings linger, shaping our thoughts, our reactions, our very sense of self. If you, like me, have found yourself feeling distant, harsh, or envious without truly understanding why—it's not because you're flawed or broken. It's because there's a part of you, a younger version of you, who is still waiting to be seen, to be appreciated, to be loved, to be healed.

Healing the Inner Child

Today, I continue the work of healing old wounds, striving to live from a place of love rather than fear. This journey has been one of the hardest but most necessary steps I've ever taken. As I reparent my inner child, I'm learning to give myself the love and validation I've always longed for. This process has allowed me to connect more authentically with others and, most importantly, with myself.

If any of this resonates with you—if you recognize these very feelings—I want you to know that you're not alone. I'm sharing this from a place of deep vulnerability because I believe no one should remain imprisoned in the shadows of their past, burdened by shame or guilt, as if their story is already written. Surviving is not the same as truly living. The wounds you carry don't have to define your future. YOU have the power to rewrite it. By acknowledging and nurturing your inner child and committing to the brave work of healing, you can begin to transform your narrative so you can fully embrace the life you were meant to live. This isn't just a possibility; it's within your reach. Embrace this journey with courage and determination and you'll discover the strength to heal, connect more deeply, and build the meaningful relationships you've always desired.

Moving Forward

We may not be able to change the past, but we can understand it, learn from it, and choose how we move forward. My hope is that, through these words, you feel the sincerity of my commitment to growing into a person who no longer lets past traumas dictate their actions.

This is a journey many of us are on—a journey to understand ourselves better, to heal, and to connect more deeply with those we love. As I walk this path, I hope to offer you not just an apology but a hand to hold as we navigate this complex process of healing together.

A Heartfelt Apology to My Inner Child

There is one person to whom I owe the deepest and most heartfelt apology: my inner child. This is the part of me that was never fully nurtured, never truly seen, growing up feeling misunderstood, judged, uncared for and unworthy. To that young girl who lived through so many lonely and painful moments, I reach out now with the utmost sincerity and love.

To my inner child, I am profoundly sorry.

You were the little girl with a bright spirit whose tender heart desperately needed the safety and protection that every child deserves. In a world that should have shielded you from harm and embraced your innocence you were left exposed and alone, yearning for the comfort and security that was so elusive. My heart aches with remorse for every moment you felt abandoned, neglected, and unprotected. You should have been enveloped in the nurturing care that would have allowed you to feel truly safe and valued. I am deeply sorry for the profound sense of insecurity you endured, the deep yearning you desired, knowing you deserved so much more than what you received.

You faced fears that you couldn't share with anyone. You carried burdens that no child should ever bear and I want you to know that there is no shame in those experiences. You didn't deserve the pain or the guilt that you felt. It was never nor will it be ever your fault. The darkness you suffered was not a reflection of your worth but the result of circumstances beyond your control.

You were never truly happy. You never fully experienced the pure joy and contentment that every child deserves. I am so sorry that you had to diminish your light, not because you wanted to but because you didn't believe you deserved anything good. Your brilliance was dimmed by the shadows of unworthiness and the burden of unmet needs. It breaks my heart to think that you were forced to hide your true self because you felt you didn't deserve to shine brightly.

If you could see me now, you would be so proud. Despite the overwhelming challenges and the times when you were convinced you couldn't continue living, you showed extraordinary bravery. Your strength, even when it felt like you had none left, has guided us to this place of healing. I see now how incredibly resilient you were and I want you to know that your courage has shaped who I am today.

After many decades of struggle and profound self-discovery, we are finally stepping into a new chapter—a chapter where the pain of the past no longer dictates the present. We used to be bound by walls made of fear and sadness, but now they have been brought down giving way to a space where you can finally be free. You are now free to dream, to laugh, to play, and to simply be. You no longer need to be defined by the hurt and neglect of your early years. You can reclaim the innocence and joy that were once out of reach.

You are now free to explore the world with a sense of wonder and playfulness that you were never allowed to experience before. This freedom is not just about escaping the past but about rediscovering the simple pleasures of life. It's time to let go of the pain and sorrow that have held you captive for so long and embrace the possibility of healing and renewal.

I am here to support you every step of the way, to help you navigate this new chapter of ours. You can trust that it's safe to let go and it's safe to be who you were always meant to be. I will always be here, ready to offer the love and care you have long deserved. You are never alone in this journey. I am committed to nurturing you, to being the parent you needed, and to providing the love, care and validation that was once unattainable.

Together, we will mend the past and welcome a future where you are cherished, valued, and loved beyond measure. You are precious, deeply loved, and worthy of all the care and kindness I can offer. At last, you may finally be who you were always intended to be—an innocent child. Let this be a new beginning, where you can truly live, laugh, and love. In this journey of healing, let's cherish each moment of growth and transformation. I am here to celebrate your resilience and to remind you daily of your inherent worth. You are a radiant light, deserving of all the joy, happiness and love this life has to offer.

With all my love and dedication,

Meeting Yourself Where You Are

Healing from unresolved trauma is a deeply personal journey, one that calls for compassion, patience, and a willingness to truly see ourselves. Each person's experience is unique and it's crucial to acknowledge where you are in your emotional landscape as you step onto this path of recovery. By tuning into your current level of consciousness—your thoughts, feelings, and overall mental state—you can find the right healing strategies that resonate with you.

We begin by cultivating self-awareness of your emotions and behaviors. Reflect on the situations, people, or memories that evoke uncomfortable feelings or reactions. Make it a habit to regularly check in with yourself to assess your emotional state. Ask questions like, "Am I feeling anxious, sad, or angry?" Understanding your feelings can provide insights into your readiness to confront unresolved issues in your life. Use simple check-in prompts such as, "What am I feeling right now?" or "What do I need at this moment?" This practice not only encourages you to connect with your emotional landscape but also guides you in addressing your needs with kindness and understanding.

CHAPTER 1

To Understand Your 'SELF', Start Here

Unresolved pain can affect every part of your life, including how you parent. Your child might sense your hesitation or the overcompensation stemming from unfulfilled needs in your past. They may absorb your unhealed wounds, even when you don't intend for them to. Holding on to this pain because you think it makes you stronger can make things worse. It festers and impacts your relationships, your joy, and your parenting.

So how do you break this cycle? The answer is as difficult as it is simple—healing. It involves the death of the old self, shedding the layers that have been defined by pain, fear, and avoidance. You confront the long-avoided corners of your mind where painful memories reside. You grieve and allow yourself to feel all the emotions—sadness, anger, joy, betrayal, loss. You can only move forward when you give yourself permission to feel, acknowledge and release these emotions, instead of letting them continue to live inside you.

Jim Rohn once said, "The greatest value in life is to serve others." Healing yourself isn't just about personal relief; it's also about the value you bring to those around you. When you address and begin to heal unresolved trauma, you're better equipped to genuinely serve your loved ones. You not only break the cycle of pain but also become a more compassionate and effective parent. In this way, your journey toward healing enriches not just your life but the lives of those you care for.

What Is IFS (Internal Family Systems)?

Whenever you say, "A part of me feels…" or "A part of me thinks…" you're often acknowledging that there are different aspects of your emotional or psychological self. It's a way of recognizing that your feelings or thoughts can be complex and that different parts of you might have different perspectives or responses. For example, you might say, "A part of me is excited about the new job opportunity, but another part of me is anxious about the change." This helps you convey the complexity of your emotions or thoughts, acknowledging that you can experience conflicting feelings or viewpoints at the same time.

Now, imagine your mind as a vibrant village, each resident representing a different part of you—some are protectors, some are critics, and others carry old wounds. These "parts" all aim to keep you safe and thriving, even if they sometimes clash and pull you in different directions. If this idea still feels abstract, consider the animated film *Inside Out* (2015), directed by Pete Docter. The story unfolds within the mind of an 11-year-old girl named Riley, where her emotions—Joy, Sadness, Anger, Fear, and Disgust—are personified as characters that influence her behavior and decisions. Each of these emotions takes the reins at different moments, vying for control based on what they think Riley needs at the time.

Much like the characters in *Inside Out*, your mind houses various "parts" that hold unique feelings, perspectives, and roles. Understanding this inner dynamic is key to uncovering the true essence of your "Self"—the calm, compassionate core of who you are. Hold on to this concept as we'll revisit it in the following chapters.

Our brains are amazing survival devices, well-calibrated to guard against damage. But in their well-meaning attempts to protect us, they can sometimes cause inner conflict, leaving us feeling stuck or overburdened. The Internal

Family Systems (IFS) model, developed by Dr. Richard Schwartz in the 1980s (Schwartz, 1995), offers a powerful framework for understanding and navigating our inner worlds. Personally, I have found IFS to be incredibly helpful in my journey, enabling me to unravel the complexities of my mind and work toward deeper self-integration.

IFS invites us to see our minds as a collection of distinct parts, much like the way *Inside Out* portrays emotions as individual characters. Each part has its own voice, memories, and goals. These parts may sometimes compete with or misunderstand one another, but they all share the same overarching goal: to protect you and ensure your well-being. By approaching your inner world with curiosity and compassion, you can begin to harmonize these voices and foster a more holistic sense of self.

Key Concepts in IFS:

The Self: This represents your core essence—who you are at your deepest level. The Self is calm, curious, and compassionate, acting as a wise leader for your internal system.

(In the context of *Inside Out*, while there isn't a specific character that represents the Self, you can think of it as the part of you that can step back, observe all your emotions or parts, and guide them with understanding and balance.)

Parts: These are the sub-personalities or facets of the self, each holding specific emotions, beliefs, and experiences. Common parts include the Manager, the Firefighter, and the Exile. Each part has its own role and can either support or hinder your well-being.

(Just as the characters in *Inside Out* each take turns steering Riley's thoughts and reactions, our internal parts influence how we navigate the world. Some parts, like Joy, act as protectors, working hard to maintain control and keep us happy. Others, like Sadness, represent the vulnerable, wounded aspects of ourselves, carrying the weight of deeper emotional pain.

In the sequel, we encounter a new set of emotions: Anxiety, Envy, and Embarrassment. Anxiety might take center stage, responding to perceived threats or uncertainties with a heightened sense of alertness. Envy could emerge as a reflection of our desires and perceived deficiencies, pushing us to confront and understand our aspirations and comparisons. Embarrassment might show up to signal when we've stepped out of our comfort zone or violated social norms, urging us to navigate social dynamics with care and self-awareness.)

Internal Dynamics: The interactions between your parts and the Self. Understanding these dynamics allows us to address internal conflicts and promote emotional healing.

(Just like in *Inside Out*, where the emotions learn to work together for Riley's well-being, IFS helps your parts collaborate under the guidance of the Self.)

How This May Look in Real Life:

Let's say you feel anxious before a big presentation. One part of you, the Manager, steps in, wanting to ensure everything goes perfectly and to prevent failure—similar to how Joy in *Inside Out* always tries to keep things upbeat. Another part, the Exile, holds on to insecurities from past experiences and doubts your abilities, much like Sadness embodies Riley's feelings of loss and uncertainty. Then there's the Firefighter, a part that might try to protect you by avoiding the situation entirely—perhaps by distracting you or encouraging procrastination, much like Fear or Disgust might react when they feel overwhelmed.

In IFS, when the Self—your calm, compassionate core—takes charge, it can reassure the Manager to prepare without becoming overbearing, comfort the Exile's insecurities, and guide the Firefighter to stay focused and present. This process of balancing and harmonizing your internal parts helps you approach challenges with more confidence and ease, just as the emotions in *Inside Out* eventually learn to work together to support Riley.

What Is Neuro-Linguistic Programming (NLP)?

While IFS focuses on understanding and harmonizing the different parts of your psyche, Neuro-Linguistic Programming (NLP) provides tools to reshape your interactions with these parts and with the world around you. Neuro-Linguistic Programming, developed in the 1970s by Richard Bandler and John Grinder, explores how our brain and nervous system react to different situations. Essentially, it examines the functions of the brain, the use of language, and how these elements influence our behavior (Bandler & Grinder, 1975).

NLP aims to help people understand and transform their thoughts and actions by examining this connection, making it especially effective in changing how you perceive and respond to life's challenges.

NLP teaches us that our subjective experience of the world is largely shaped by our internal language—the words and mental images we use to describe our experiences. By understanding and modifying this internal language we can change our emotional states, behaviors, and even beliefs.

Key Concepts in NLP:

Anchoring: This is a technique where a specific stimulus (like a touch, sound, or word) is used to trigger a particular emotional state. Anchors can help you quickly access positive states of mind, which is particularly useful when working with challenging internal parts in IFS.

Submodalities: These are the finer distinctions within our sensory experiences (like brightness in visual images or volume in sounds). By altering submodalities, you can change how you perceive and feel about different memories or situations, making it easier to work with difficult parts.

Reframing: This involves changing the context or perspective of a situation to alter its meaning. Reframing can be a powerful tool in IFS, helping you to see your parts not as obstacles but as allies with positive intentions.

Powerful Duo

By combining IFS and NLP you can create a more comprehensive approach to healing and self-development. Here's how they work together:

- **Healing Unresolved Trauma:** IFS helps you access and heal the wounded parts of you that are holding on to traumatic memories. NLP can then assist in reshaping the way these memories are stored and perceived, reducing their emotional impact and creating new, empowering narratives.

- **Enhancing Self-Communication:** IFS encourages dialogue between your parts and your Self, while NLP provides the tools to make this communication more effective. For instance, using NLP anchoring can help you maintain a state of calm (the Self) when engaging with a difficult part.

- **Rewriting Internal Narratives:** Through IFS you understand the motivations of your internal parts. NLP can help you reframe these motivations, changing the internal narrative from one of conflict to one of cooperation and growth.

The Role of IFS and NLP in Healing Childhood Trauma

IFS is especially effective in addressing childhood trauma because it helps identify and work with the parts of you that have held on to past wounds. By recognizing and validating these parts you can start to heal from trauma and develop healthier coping mechanisms.

NLP complements this by offering tools to reshape how these traumas are stored in your mind. For example, if a particular memory is strongly associated with a sense of fear, NLP techniques can help diminish the intensity of that fear, making it easier to work with that memory in IFS.

A Non-Pathologizing Approach

Approaching this journey with a non-pathologizing mindset is crucial. Instead of viewing your inner parts as problems to be fixed, see them as adaptations that were once necessary for your survival. Throughout the book, you will be encouraged to view these parts not as flaws but as responses to past experiences. You will also be empowered with tools to reframe these experiences, allowing you to view them from a position of strength and learning.

We'll focus on understanding and integrating these parts without judgment. Each part of you has a role and a reason for its behavior. By treating them with curiosity and kindness, and by applying these techniques to enhance understanding, you can create a dialogue that leads to healing and personal growth.

How IFS and NLP Will Be Integrated Throughout This Book

You will come across a variety of ideas and activities in this book that have their roots in both NLP and IFS. Gaining knowledge of these concepts will improve how you relate to the information and apply it to your life. Here's how they will be integrated:

- **Interactive Exercises:** These will include prompts for exploring your internal parts (IFS) and applying NLP techniques to reshape how you perceive and interact with these parts.

- **Self-Assessments:** Tools for assessing your internal dynamics (IFS) will help identify which parts are most active in your life, while NLP will help you modify these dynamics for more positive outcomes.

- **Healing Strategies:** Modalities for therapeutic healing will be informed by both IFS and NLP principles, guiding you to work with your internal parts and reframe your experiences to achieve greater emotional balance and resilience.

Getting Started with IFS and NLP

To begin integrating IFS and NLP into your journey, let's reflect on these questions:

1. What parts of you do you notice most frequently? Are there specific emotions or behaviors that seem to dominate your experience?

2. How do these parts interact with one another? Do you notice any internal conflicts or recurring patterns in your life?

3. What role does your Self play in guiding your internal system? How connected do you feel to your core essence?

4. How does your internal language shape your experience of these parts? Are there any narratives or beliefs that you'd like to reframe?

By exploring these questions and engaging with IFS and NLP concepts, you'll lay a strong foundation for the rest of the book. The insights you gain will support your journey toward healing and personal transformation.

I encourage you to be persistent and patient. The greater part of this journey will be pleasant, profoundly touching. However, growth occurs in cycles of activity and rest. In the beginning, you may feel like you're making great strides, but later on, you might feel like you're stuck and not making much progress. Or you can experience an accelerated pace of your inner growth, leaving you feeling as if you're slipping back. You may sometimes discover that a problem you believed you had handled has returned more powerfully than before. This simply signifies that you have exposed this particular "enemy" for control or defeat. Other times, an unpleasant sensation from the past comes back, which only signals that you're ready to experience and heal deeply.

"Smell of Fresh Paint"

I was four, going on five, when my mom and I moved into a new apartment. The smell of fresh paint was still in the air, marking the start of something new. I remember the mix of excitement and uncertainty, with everything around me feeling both familiar and strange. Yet, there was also a profound sense of relief and an almost indescribable feeling of safety, even though I didn't fully understand what "safe" meant at that age. I clearly recall the thrill of having a birthday party in the new place and the excitement of going to watch *Disney on Ice* the very same day. It was a time of new beginnings, one filled with joy and wonder. But even with all the fun, there was something much heavier that stood out from that time.

A relative came over one late afternoon and I remember watching from the stairs, peeking through the gaps between the steps. What began as a casual visit quickly escalated into a heated argument. The voices grew louder, more intense, as they moved from friendly chatter about our new home and furniture to heated demands for money. The yelling and screaming got so loud that I was sure the neighbors could hear every word.

I clung to the wooden railing, trying to make myself as small as possible. I was only five years old, so I didn't really understand what was going on with them, but I could feel the tension, that something was off. I remember feeling embarrassed and scared, acutely aware of the neighbors' eyes that might be peeking through their windows, witnessing the chaos. The thought of them judging us, this new family in the neighborhood, made my stomach knot even tighter.

As the visitor finally stormed out, the house felt different—like the anger had seeped into the walls along with the smell of fresh paint. I watched my mother as she slumped into a chair, her face a mask of exhaustion and sadness. Even then, I began to understand, in my small way, that she was carrying a burden far heavier than I could comprehend. And somehow, without knowing it, I found myself carrying a piece of that burden with her. In hindsight, that was the first time I recognized the emotional burden my mother was carrying. It was invisible but undeniably real, something she'd been carrying long before that argument. As the years passed, I became more attuned to this weight she never seemed to put down. Mothers throughout the world carry this "invisible load," a weight that often begins in their own childhoods and continues through the years, sometimes unnoticed, sometimes overwhelming. And as children, we pick up on these things, feeling responsible for the emotions of those we love, even when we're too young to fully grasp what's happening. It's a burden that shapes us in ways we might not understand until much later in life. And so an empath is born.

CHAPTER 2

The Invisible Load of Motherhood

You're juggling a toddler on the brink of a grocery store meltdown while your phone incessantly buzzes with urgent work emails and a mountain of laundry waits at home that is threatening to avalanche. You're mentally ticking off dinner plans, stressing over a dentist appointment you nearly forgot, and wondering if you ever RSVP'd to that birthday party that barely fits into your packed schedule. And just when you think you've got a handle on things, you remember the school volunteering commitment, the kids' marching band practice, the chicken still frozen in the freezer, and the cycling class you're supposed to teach later. Sound familiar?

Studies show that the average mother manages an enormous mental load, often referred to as the "invisible load." This burden includes not only the logistics of daily life but also the emotional labor involved in keeping a family functioning smoothly. According to a study by Ciciolla and Luthar (2019) published in *Sex Roles*, invisible household labor significantly affects mothers' psychological adjustment.

We moms often bear this invisible burden—a relentless mental and emotional to-do list that seems to grow no matter how much we handle. This isn't just about managing household chaos and endless errands; it's about the unyielding pressure to stay ahead, to keep everything running smoothly while balancing emotional labor and societal expectations. This load that you can't see is heavy, often thankless, constant, and never truly letting up.

Yet, through it all, you're always there, making sure your little ones feel loved and cared for. It's like imaginary spinning plates—dinner, school projects, work deadlines, and self-care (what's that?)—with your mind on autopilot updating the to-do list without an "off" switch. I understand the challenges of managing multiple responsibilities and the sense of being overwhelmed and sometimes feeling undervalued.

I remember a time when all the kids were down with a stomach flu. Details aside, I felt defeated as I did everything I could to comfort them while teetering on the edge of exhaustion, worry and, yes, frustration. I'd wake up with puffy eyes, looking like I cried through the night—because, well, I did. To add more nonsense, I also convinced myself I'd never measure up to those moms who seemed to have it all together, showing off their kids' perfectly fishtail-braided hair on Instagram. But here's what I've learned: simply getting up the next day, even when you're hanging by a thread, is proof of just how incredibly resilient we are as mothers. Yes, it's hard; yes it's challenging, but because we love so, so deeply we find all the courage we can muster to keep going.

The weight you carry isn't just heavy. It's all-consuming. The mental and emotional load, along with societal expectations, can take a toll on your health. According to the American Psychological Association, chronic stress from managing multiple roles can lead to burnout and health issues like anxiety and depression. It becomes even more disheartening when your hard work is unnoticed or undervalued. However, you press on with perseverance and that is nothing short of amazing. Don't you forget it!

"A Mother's Silent Ally"

Once upon a time, in a world where emotions and physical sensations could speak, there was a mother named Dawn. Like other moms, she found herself overwhelmed by the daily demands of life, juggling work, family, and endless responsibilities. Each day felt like an exhausting marathon and she often felt as if she was running on empty.

If her body could talk, it would have said, "I'm on your side, not working against you! I'm here in ways you might not even recognize. I'm the one showing you where your limits lie, expressing them through the aches and stresses that you feel when you push yourself too hard. I'm the tiredness that often lingers, the weariness you brush aside because you think you don't have time to rest."

Dawn often dismissed her headaches, moments of brain fog, and occasional stomach ache, chalking them up to being just another part of motherhood. But deep down, her body was sending out a desperate call for help. "Please, listen to me!" it would plead. "These signs aren't just annoyances; they're my way of reminding you to pay attention to what you truly need. You're doing so much for everyone else, but you also deserve care and rest!"

One evening, after a particularly chaotic day of juggling school pickups, work deadlines, and dinner preparations, Dawn collapsed onto her bed. As she lay there, she closed her eyes and took a deep breath, allowing the weight of her exhaustion to wash over her. In that moment of stillness, she could almost hear her body whispering, "I'm here for you. Remember, taking care of yourself isn't selfish; it's essential. You can't pour from an empty cup."

That night, Dawn made a promise to herself. She would start listening—to the gentle nudges and urgent pleas of her body. She would take moments to rest, set boundaries, and allow herself the grace she readily offered others. As she began to honor her own needs, she discovered a new rhythm in her life, one that filled her with renewed energy and clarity. One that allow her to embrace the beautiful chaos of motherhood with a little more joy and a lot more strength.

The Subtle Signs of Overactive Stress

1. **Emotional Drain**: An overactive stress response can make minor interactions feel overwhelming. You might find yourself snapping at loved ones or withdrawing from social activities. Recognizing these patterns helps you understand how stress affects your relationships.

2. **Physical Symptoms**: Stress often manifests in physical symptoms like headaches, muscle tension, or digestive issues. These symptoms are your body's way of communicating that it's overworked. Paying attention to these signs can help you address your underlying stressors.

3. **Difficulty Enjoying Life**: If stress is making it hard to savor simple, joyful moments, it's not just about feeling overwhelmed; it's about how stress robs you of your ability to experience happiness fully. Identifying and reclaiming these moments can be a powerful step in healing.

4. **Constant Exhaustion**: Feeling perpetually drained isn't just about physical tiredness; it's your body's way of signaling that stress is depleting your energy reserves. If you're constantly running on empty, it might be worth exploring how stress contributes to your fatigue.

5. **Sleep Disturbances**: Struggling with insomnia or disrupted sleep patterns is a common sign of stress. Whether it's trouble falling asleep, staying asleep, or waking up too early, stress can significantly

impact the quality of your rest, further affecting your overall well-being. We'll talk more in coming chapters about the solutions to this.

6. **Frequent Illness**: Catching colds or experiencing other illnesses can be a sign that your immune system is compromised. When you're under chronic stress, your body's ability to fight off infections can diminish, which makes you more susceptible to illnesses.

Future-Proofing Your Recovery from Trauma

As a mother with unresolved trauma, your healing journey is deeply personal, but it requires tools and strategies that can support you not just today but more so in the future. To truly heal and grow you need a plan that evolves with you—one that empowers you to make choices that nurture your well-being and resilience over time.

Here's how to future-proof your recovery, ensuring you build a foundation for lasting wellness and growth:

1. Understanding Trauma and Its Impact on You

Empirical evidence shows that trauma affects not only your emotional well-being but also your physical health and relationships. Recognizing how trauma manifests in your life—whether through stress, anxiety, or difficulty connecting with others—is the first step toward building a sustainable healing process.

2. Empowering Strategies to Take Control

In the upcoming chapters, we'll dive into specific strategies to help you take control of your stress response. You'll learn techniques to identify stress patterns, create mini-rituals for daily relief, reframe your perspective, build a supportive network, and practice self-compassion. While circumstances may contribute to your stress, remember that you are not a product of your circumstances—you are a product of your choices. By consciously managing stress you can improve your health and life balance. These strategies will empower you to thrive not only now but in the long term.

3. Building Flexibility into Your Healing

Healing from trauma is not a linear process. Different methods, like mindfulness practices, therapy, or self-compassion exercises, may work at different stages of your journey. The key to future-proofing your recovery is allowing for flexibility. As you grow and change so should your approach to healing. Be open to adjusting your methods and finding new ways to care for yourself as your needs evolve.

4. Cultivating Resilience for the Future

Research shows that resilience—the ability to bounce back from difficult emotions and life challenges—is essential to long-term recovery. Building resilience doesn't happen overnight, but it can be nurtured through small, consistent practices like setting boundaries, managing stress, and embracing self-care. These are lifelong skills that will not only help you heal but also set a powerful example for your children.

5. Creating a Support Network That Lasts

You don't have to walk this path alone. Whether it's connecting with other moms, joining support groups, or seeking professional guidance, having a network of ongoing support is crucial to future-proofing your recovery. As you continue to heal these relationships will provide you with strength and encouragement, ensuring that you always have a safe space to turn to, even as life changes.

6. **Honoring Your Individual Path**

Your trauma, your story, and your needs are unique to you. As you move forward remember that your healing journey will look different from anyone else's. By honoring your own pace, finding what works best for you, and being kind to yourself along the way you create a future-proofed path to long-term wellness.

By focusing on future-proofing your recovery through empowering strategies and adaptable tools you'll not only heal from your trauma but also build a lasting foundation for growth, strength, and resilience. In the chapters ahead, we will equip you with the techniques to consciously shape your well-being and thrive both for yourself and for your family.

Embrace the Power of Small Victories

Imagine someone offered you an enormous amount of money, more than you could ever spend, but accepting it would mean giving up something far more valuable: the everyday moments that define your life as a mother. No amount of money could ever replace the worth of your love, the tiny victories you achieve each day, and the unique role you play in your family's life.

As a mother, your life is incredibly valuable! Every small victory—whether it's managing a busy morning, finding those elusive matching socks, or simply making it through a challenging day—is no easy feat. These moments might seem small, inconsequential, and are easy to overlook because of their everyday nature. But they highlight your ability to navigate life's demands with grace and unwavering commitment, even when tasks feel repetitive or mundane.

It's easy to feel like the work you do as a mother is monotonous so you minimize its significance. The daily routine can make it hard to see the bigger picture. But if you take it too lightly, these moments will slip by unnoticed. Just now, while writing this, I had a conversation with one of my kids. They told me they wanted to leave the country to attend school. The realization hit me hard—one day you're helping them glue their "100th day" project in kinder and the next you're scouting apartments in a different country.

You've probably heard people say, "Time flies," and it truly does. One day you're pushing strollers, maybe even finding yourself complain how you just vacuumed the car and it's dirty again, and next you're helping them fill out college applications. It's in those small moments that you realize how quickly they grow and how each seemingly insignificant day contributes to their journey.

The truth is your impact is enormous. Just as you pour love and care into your family, it's just as vital to take a moment to acknowledge your own contributions. Recognizing these small victories isn't just a nice gesture—it's a way to nurture yourself and sustain your well-being as you parent with unshakeable confidence.

You play an extraordinary role in your family's life and even the smallest wins deserve to be celebrated. Appreciate these everyday successes because you're investing in your own happiness and health. Each step forward (or backwards), no matter how small, is part of the beautiful journey of motherhood. So embrace your achievements with warmth and pride, knowing that you deserve all the joy and fulfillment this path has to offer.

Emotional Check-In:

Take a moment to pause and check in with yourself. So, how does reading this make you feel? Feeling a bit overwhelmed? That's okay. Just remember, you're not alone in this. We all go through tough times. I see you. Just take a moment to breathe, my friend, and let's tackle that hidden burden together.

Think about how this load impacts not only your day-to-day existence but also your overall health and relationships.

Think back to those times when you really felt the weight of this invisible burden. Have you noticed any changes in how you interact with your family or how you feel about yourself? It's important to be aware of these emotions as the initial step in discovering helpful strategies to handle and lighten this weight.

Being a mom is far more than a role—it's a calling and you embody it with strength, grace, and wisdom that often go unspoken. You are not "just a mom"—you are the steady force behind your family's success, the one who keeps everything running, even when no one is watching. Your work is profound, your love is boundless, and your dedication shapes the very foundation of those you care for. Every action, no matter how small, contributes to the life and happiness of your family and that is nothing short of remarkable.

The Overlooked Brilliance behind Motherhood

Here's a glimpse into the incredible qualities that you demonstrate every single day:

Unwavering Dedication
Your consistent effort and commitment to managing both visible and hidden responsibilities show an incredible dedication to your family's well-being.

Exceptional Organizational Skills
Balancing multiple tasks simultaneously reflects your extraordinary ability to organize and manage a complex household efficiently.

Creative Problem-Solving
Handling unexpected challenges and finding solutions to daily issues demonstrate your creativity and resourcefulness in making things work smoothly.

Deep Emotional Intelligence
The constant mental and emotional juggling reveals a profound understanding and empathy toward your family's needs and feelings.

Remarkable Resilience
The ability to keep going, even when the load feels overwhelming, showcases your resilience and inner strength, adapting to changing circumstances.

Hidden Acts of Love
The unnoticed efforts, like planning and remembering special moments, reflect your deep love and commitment to creating a nurturing environment.

Masterful Multitasking
Managing various responsibilities with grace highlights your ability to multitask effectively, balancing numerous aspects of family life seamlessly.

Unseen Nurturing
The care and attention given to maintaining a harmonious home, even if not always visible, underscores your nurturing role in fostering a supportive family environment.

Invisible Contributions to Stability
The quiet, ongoing efforts that contribute to the family's overall stability and happiness reveal your crucial role in keeping everything running smoothly.

Selfless Sacrifice
The often overlooked sacrifices made for the sake of your family's needs and happiness showcase your selflessness and dedication.

These qualities make you not just the heart of your home but an extraordinary leader, nurturer, and inspiration to those around you. You deserve to be recognized, not only for what you do but for who you are—a pillar of strength, love, and wisdom. You are NOT just a mom.

Interactive Exercise:

Write Down Your Load: Grab a notebook or open a new document on your computer. Write down everything that's on your mind right now and don't hold back—every worry, every task, every "should." This could include things like meal planning, doctor's appointments, deadlines, or even the pressure to maintain a clean house and get every crumb between the sofa cushions (yes, I'm looking at you, hidden snacks).

Once you've listed everything, take a moment to reflect on the weight of this list. Which items are most pressing? Which ones can you delegate or let go of? Remember, this isn't about whether each item "sparks joy" like Marie Kondo would have you believe; it's about whether they're necessary to your sanity. Does the pantry really need to be reorganized again? Today?

Inhale deeply and tell yourself that even Marie sometimes lets a few crumbs fall between the gaps.

To evaluate where your mental energy is going, try sorting your list into categories like job, family, and personal. You may use this to prioritize what really requires your attention and spot trends.

Next Steps:

Before you move on to the next chapter, I want you to try something. Look at your list and pick just one thing to focus on. Maybe it's setting aside time to tackle a specific task or deciding to let something go. We'll tackle the rest later, but starting with one manageable item can help ease the feeling of being overwhelmed.

Make a commitment to yourself to address this one item and notice how it impacts your stress levels. Small, actionable steps can create a ripple effect of positive change, making the overall load feel more manageable.

"A Price Too High To Pay"

My memories of time spent with both of my parents together are rare and fragmented. I remember one afternoon, coming out of a movie theater, and it was darker than usual—strangely so. People around us were holding up umbrellas, but it wasn't raining. I was confused. My mom handed me a handkerchief to cover my face, mentioning something about ashes falling from the sky.

This was during the time Mount Pinatubo erupted in 1991, the second-largest volcanic eruption of the 20th century. The ashfall blanketed large parts of the Philippines, and while I didn't fully understand it then, it sure left a lasting impression on me. It was a strange, almost apocalyptic moment when the natural world mirrored the uncertainty I felt as a child.

Around this time, my mother had come back to vacation from working abroad as a nanny. I was so happy to have her home with us—those rare moments of togetherness felt like precious gifts. But even in my joy I knew she couldn't stay for long. Soon, she would have to return to the job that had taken her away from us in the first place. The warmth of having her near was always shadowed by the sadness of knowing she would leave again. Much like the ash falling from the sky, that feeling lingered—both familiar and troubling, reminding me how fragile and temporary some things could be but also how permanent some of these "things" could be.

Later in life, what stood out more vividly were the deeply unsettling moments from my younger childhood. It was in the early '80s when my parents decided to move to the Middle East in search of a better life and I was left behind with relatives. There are particular memories that stick with me from this time—moments when I felt the distance between us acutely and the confusion of a world that felt unfamiliar. While they were building a future abroad, I was left to navigate the changes, just like I had navigated those ashes falling from the sky.

The family members who took care of me during that period were intermittent, if not often absent, and I found myself frequently watched over by neighbors they trusted. These neighbors, who were supposed to provide stability and care, instead became sources of betrayal. As a young child, I was naive, unable to fully understand the complexities or dangers of these situations. I felt abandoned and vulnerable and I struggled with emotions too big for me to express.

As I grew older and began to remember those moments, the sense of violation became painfully clear. I realized how my boundaries as a very young child had been crossed. But as a toddler, how could I have known what was acceptable or not? That it was more than simply a harmless game of hide and seek. The realization of these breaches of trust was excruciating. My innocent understanding of safety and security had been shattered, which left emotional scars that festered and took decades to fully comprehend.

I understand that my parents' decision to move away was driven by their desire to provide a better future for me. Although their departure was incredibly heartbreaking for me, I recognize it was motivated by love and hope for improved opportunities. I don't place blame on them; instead, I see their actions as a reflection of their deep care and the difficult choices they faced.

The sense of abandonment and betrayal I felt is a stark reminder of how formative these early years are. It highlights the profound effect that early trauma can have on our development and our ability to confidently trust those around us. It underscores the importance of acknowledging and healing from these early wounds, not just for ourselves but for the well-being of our own children.

I see how these experiences shaped my understanding of relationships and trust, or lack of. They influenced how I navigated my interactions with others and how I approached motherhood. For those of you who have faced similar challenges, know that you are not alone. Recognizing and addressing these wounds will be a crucial step towards your healing so you too can begin to foster a nurturing environment for your own children.

CHAPTER 3

The Baggage I Didn't Know I Had

To understand how unresolved trauma influences our lives it is useful to consider **Maslow's Hierarchy of Needs**. Developed by psychologist **Abraham Maslow** in 1943, this theory outlines a framework for understanding human motivation and personal development. Maslow proposed that human needs are arranged in a hierarchical structure, often depicted as a pyramid with five levels.

At the base of the pyramid are **physiological needs**, such as food, water, warmth, and rest—these are the fundamental requirements for survival. Once these basic needs are met, individuals can focus on the next level, **safety needs**, which include security and stability in one's environment, such as personal safety, financial security, and health.

The third level encompasses **belongingness and love needs**, where social relationships, friendships, and emotional connections become essential. Humans are inherently social beings and the need for love and acceptance plays a significant role in our emotional well-being.

Moving up the hierarchy, we encounter **esteem needs**, which involve the desire for self-esteem and recognition from others. This level reflects our need for accomplishment, respect, and validation in both personal and professional contexts.

Finally, at the top of the pyramid is **self-actualization**, the process of realizing one's full potential and pursuing personal growth. This includes creative expression, achieving goals, and finding purpose in life.

Maslow's Hierarchy serves as a valuable tool for understanding how trauma can disrupt this progression. When unresolved trauma impacts our sense of safety or belonging, it creates barriers that hinder our ability to meet higher-level needs. By examining this framework we can gain insight into the ways trauma affects our lives and the paths we can take toward healing and fulfillment.

Maslow's Hierarchy of Needs is often depicted as a pyramid with the following five levels:

1. Physiological Needs:
These are the basic survival necessities that must be met first.

- Access to food and water to stay nourished and hydrated.
- A mother ensures her family has healthy meals and a safe, comfortable place for her and her children to rest.

2. Safety Needs:
Once physiological needs are met, individuals seek security and protection from harm.

- Looking for job security to ensure a steady income and financial stability.
- A mother seeks a stable home and a safe environment for her children, including finding good childcare or schools.

3. Love and Belongingness Needs:

This level emphasizes the importance of social relationships and feeling connected to others.

- Building close friendships and maintaining family connections provide emotional support and a sense of belonging.
- A mother creates strong bonds with her children and partner while also finding support in relationships with other moms or family members.

4. Esteem Needs:

At this level, individuals strive for self-respect, recognition, and a sense of accomplishment.

- Receiving praise at work for completing a project boosts self-esteem and recognition.
- A mother feels proud and validated when her efforts in raising her children are acknowledged, like when her kids do well in school or express love and appreciation.

5. Self-Actualization:

At the top of the pyramid, individuals focus on personal growth, self-fulfillment, and realizing their full potential.

- Pursuing a passion, such as learning a new skill, starting a business, or traveling the world.
- A mother pursues personal dreams beyond parenting, such as going back to school, starting a side business, or finding fulfillment in hobbies that nurture her sense of self.

"Soleil & Luna: The Art of Procrastination"

In 2020, when the pandemic brought the world to a standstill, I launched Soleil & Luna, an event pop-up company. The idea emerged from my deep desire to create meaningful experiences during a time when connection felt scarce. It seemed like the perfect venture, filled with promise and purpose, especially amid uncertainty. What I didn't realize then was that Soleil & Luna was more than just a business—it was my way of coping with the internal chaos that the pandemic had magnified.

Initially, the excitement of starting something new fueled my energy. I immersed myself in every detail, working tirelessly to ensure its success. However, as the initial thrill faded, crippling exhaustion set in. The burnout became overwhelming and I began to lose the joy and passion that had once driven me. Looking back, I can see that Soleil & Luna was never really about the business itself; it was an attempt to distract myself from unresolved trauma amplified by the pandemic's isolation and uncertainty.

Maslow's hierarchy of needs suggests that once we meet our lower-level needs—such as safety, belonging, and self-esteem—we can only focus on higher-level goals like personal achievement (Maslow, 1943). For me, those foundational needs had been disrupted long before the pandemic due to early and severe trauma; yet, I was still trying to pursue lofty goals like entrepreneurship and personal success. Without addressing the deeper issues, I was constantly fighting an uphill battle. At the time, I couldn't see that my unresolved trauma was a barrier to truly thriving, no matter how hard I worked or how much I wanted it.

In many ways, procrastination became my way of avoiding the deeper emotional work I needed to do. When faced with overwhelming unresolved trauma, it's easy to subconsciously delay addressing those foundational needs by diverting our attention to less pressing tasks or lofty ambitions (Sirois, 2014). For me, Soleil & Luna became a form of avoidance—a way to feel "productive and successful" without facing the uncomfortable emotions beneath the surface. It provided temporary relief but ultimately stalled my personal growth and fulfillment.

What I didn't understand at the time was that my procrastination wasn't laziness or a lack of discipline; it was a coping mechanism. It allowed me to delay confronting my trauma, even though it hindered my ability to reach my true potential. Had I recognized that procrastination stems from a desire to evade unresolved issues, I might have understood the importance and need of addressing those foundational concerns first.

Another business venture that was short-lived. Burnout overtook me and I couldn't sustain the energy to keep pushing forward. What I thought was exhaustion from overwork was really the weight of unresolved trauma pulling me down and no amount of effort or ambition could fix that. The more I pushed the clearer it became that success, in any form, would remain elusive until I prioritized my healing.

Why am I sharing this? I've learned the hard way that unresolved trauma compromises our lower needs, especially those related to safety, belonging, and self-esteem, making it challenging (but not impossible) to pursue higher-level goals like success, personal achievement, or self-actualization. It's tempting to believe we can power through and achieve our dreams without confronting the pain we carry, but that only leads to burnout and frustration.

In my case, the result was a painful and avoidable failure. If I had recognized sooner that I needed to confront my trauma and rebuild my foundation, I could have spared myself the exhaustion and heartbreak of watching my business fade. It's not just about avoiding failure; it's about realizing that healing must come first. Only by addressing those core issues can we build something truly lasting—something that won't crumble under the weight of unhealed wounds.

Understanding this has changed how I approach everything. Procrastination is no longer a tool for avoiding discomfort but a signal that something deeper needs my attention. I've come to realize that investing time and energy into healing isn't a distraction from success; it's the key to it.

The Dual Nature of Trauma: Disruption and Resilience

Safety Needs: Trauma can profoundly impact an individual's sense of security and safety. When someone experiences trauma, particularly through abuse, violence, or significant loss, their perception of safety is often compromised. This can lead to chronic anxiety, hypervigilance, or a persistent sense of danger, making it difficult for them to achieve a stable and secure environment. Without a sense of safety, addressing higher-level needs becomes a secondary concern.

Complementary Perspective: However, it is important to recognize that not all individuals are permanently stuck in this state. Many trauma survivors exhibit resilience and are able to regain a sense of safety through therapeutic interventions and support systems. Techniques like Cognitive Behavioral Therapy (CBT) and Eye Movement Desensitization and Reprocessing (EMDR) can help individuals process trauma and restore their sense of security (Shapiro, 2017). Additionally, some survivors report positive psychological growth, finding strength and appreciation for life after trauma (Tedeschi & Calhoun, 2004). This highlights that while trauma disrupts safety initially, healing and growth are possible.

Belonging and Love Needs: Trauma can extend its effects into the realm of relationships and social connections. Individuals with unresolved trauma may struggle with trust, emotional intimacy, and forming meaningful relationships. These challenges can hinder their ability to establish a supportive network or feel a sense of belonging. The disruption in social connections and the inability to experience love and acceptance can significantly impact emotional well-being, preventing progress toward fulfilling higher-level needs.

Complementary Perspective: At the same time, many trauma survivors find ways to rebuild relationships and trust over time. With effective therapy and community support individuals can work through trust issues and reconnect with others. Cultural and social factors play a significant role in this process. In collectivist societies, for example, individuals may experience stronger social support systems that help mitigate the social isolation often caused by trauma (Ng & Wong, 2012). Moreover, many survivors experience post-traumatic growth where overcoming adversity leads to deeper, more meaningful relationships and a renewed sense of belonging (Tedeschi & Calhoun, 2004). So, while trauma can disrupt social connections, it is not necessarily permanent or insurmountable.

Esteem Needs: Trauma can erode an individual's self-esteem and self-worth. Many trauma survivors struggle with feelings of inadequacy, guilt, or shame, which undermine their sense of accomplishment and recognition. Persistent negative self-perceptions can make it difficult to pursue goals or gain the recognition they seek, hindering the fulfillment of esteem needs.

Complementary Perspective: Despite this, research shows that individuals can rebuild their self-esteem over time, especially with the help of therapeutic approaches that focus on changing negative self-perceptions. In fact, some people emerge from traumatic experiences with a stronger sense of purpose and self-worth through the process of meaning-making (Park, 2010). By reframing their trauma and finding personal meaning in their experiences, survivors can rebuild their esteem and pursue new goals, demonstrating that trauma need not permanently inhibit the fulfillment of esteem needs.

Self-Actualization: Self-actualization, which involves realizing one's full potential and pursuing personal growth, can be significantly obstructed by unresolved trauma. The emotional and psychological energy consumed by trauma often overshadows efforts to engage in self-improvement or personal development. As a result, individuals may feel preoccupied with unresolved issues, making it difficult to engage in activities that lead to self-fulfillment.

Complementary Perspective: Yet, some survivors of trauma have reported that their experiences, while challenging, served as a catalyst for self-actualization. The process of overcoming trauma can foster deep introspection, encouraging individuals to pursue meaningful goals and personal growth. Viktor Frankl's work on finding meaning in suffering demonstrates how trauma can lead individuals to achieve self-actualization despite, or even because of, their experiences (Frankl, 1984). This suggests that while trauma initially disrupts self-actualization, it can also inspire survivors to seek greater purpose and growth in their lives.

Adapting Maslow's Hierarchy: Maslow's hierarchy of needs suggests that individuals must satisfy lower-level needs, like safety and belonging, before progressing to higher needs such as self-esteem and self-actualization. However, research indicates that this progression is not always linear. Maslow himself later acknowledged that individuals might pursue self-actualization even when lower-level needs remain unmet (Maslow, 1968). This flexibility suggests that while trauma may disrupt basic needs like safety or belonging, individuals can still pursue self-actualization by adapting to their circumstances and seeking growth through adversity.

Trauma undeniably disrupts an individual's ability to fulfill key psychological needs including safety, belonging, esteem, and self-actualization. However, it is essential to recognize that this disruption is not always permanent. Resilience, therapeutic interventions, cultural support systems, and the potential for post-traumatic growth demonstrate that healing is possible.

As you navigate your own journey, remember that many trauma survivors have found ways to rebuild their sense of security, reconnect with others, restore self-esteem, and achieve self-actualization. For instance, Maya Angelou, who faced childhood trauma from sexual abuse and racism, went on to become a celebrated poet and civil rights activist. Through her writing and activism she transformed her pain into powerful messages of hope and empowerment, inspiring countless individuals to rise above their circumstances.

Similarly, Viktor Frankl, a Holocaust survivor, experienced unimaginable suffering in concentration camps. He emerged not only to tell his story but also to develop a psychological approach known as Logotherapy, which emphasizes finding meaning in suffering. His book, *Man's Search for Meaning*, illustrates how even in the darkest situations individuals can discover purpose and hope (Frankl, 1984).

Oprah Winfrey is another profound example of resilience. Growing up in poverty and facing abuse and trauma, Oprah overcame immense challenges to become a media mogul and philanthropist. Her experiences fueled her desire to inspire others and through her talk show and charitable work she has touched millions of lives, advocating for education, self-improvement, and emotional healing. Oprah's story exemplifies how trauma can motivate individuals to create positive change in their own lives and the lives of others.

As someone who experienced various forms of abuse—emotional, sexual and psychological—as a child, I deeply understand the profound impact trauma can have on one's sense of self and perception of the world. Back in 2021, during the depths of my depression, if you had told me that I would one day soon be a published author, establish my podcast "Baggage: Claimed" and become a speaker, I would have laughed in disbelief. In that dark time, I had to confront the uncomfortable truth: I wasn't okay. The idea of achieving anything felt distant and unattainable. However, through perseverance, a genuine willingness to acknowledge my struggles, and the unwavering love and support of my family, I gradually found the strength to confront my past and transform my experiences into something meaningful.

In this journey, I discovered my true purpose: to be a fearless voice for resilient women and mothers alike—those who have felt silenced, dismissed, and invisible, their voices drowned out by doubt and fear, their experiences trivialized and overlooked. I want to amplify your invaluable cries for help, shining a heartfelt light on your stories and reminding you that you are not alone in this fight. This work is much bigger than me; it encompasses a collective struggle for those whose stories often go unheard. I am committed to being a voice for women like you, to illuminate your experiences and to foster a sense of community where you can find strength in shared stories. This advocacy is a mission that transcends my personal narrative, reaching toward a vision of empowerment and resilience that I could never have imagined.

The path to recovery may be challenging, but it can also lead to profound personal growth and renewed purpose. Embrace the possibility that your experiences, while painful, can serve as a catalyst for transformation. By actively engaging in your healing process and seeking the support you need you can rewrite your narrative and reclaim your sense of self.

You are not defined by your trauma but by your ability to rise above it. As you move forward in this book, give yourself the permission to explore the tools and strategies that will help facilitate your growth and well-being. Your journey is uniquely yours and within it lies the potential for renewal and hope. Remember, healing is not linear; it is a dynamic process that unfolds over time. Embrace it with an open heart, knowing that every effort you make brings you closer to a more fulfilled and meaningful life.

[TAKE A DEEP BREATH. Inhale for four, slowly exhale for six. I know we're unpacking a lot so take the time you need.

Deep breathing is a simple yet effective practice that promotes relaxation and well-being. By focusing on slow, deep breaths, individuals can activate the body's relaxation response, reducing anxiety and enhancing mood (Perciavalle et al., 2016; Brown & Gerbarg, 2013). Even a few minutes of deep breathing can help alleviate stress and restore mental clarity.]

Understanding Unresolved Trauma

"According to the *Diagnostic and Statistical Manual of Mental Disorders, 5th Edition (DSM-5)*, trauma is defined as when an individual person is exposed 'to actual or threatened death, serious injury, or sexual violence' (American Psychiatric Association [APA], 2013, p. 271)."

"**Trauma** results from an event, series of events, or set of circumstances that is experienced by an individual as physically or emotionally harmful or threatening and that has lasting adverse effects on the individual's functioning and physical, social, emotional, or spiritual well-being" (Substance Abuse and Mental Health Services Administration [SAMHSA], **Trauma** and Justice Strategic Initiative, 2012, p. 2).

Trauma is a deeply distressing experience that overwhelms our ability to cope. It is not merely an event; rather, it fragments our inner world into different "parts," with each part carrying its own burdens, memories, and emotions. These parts, central to Internal Family Systems (IFS) therapy, are like an invisible backpack filled with stones—each representing a painful memory or unresolved issue that gets heavier as time passes. This weight subtly affects our decisions, relationships, and sense of self.

Trauma is deeply embedded and it shapes our thoughts and behaviors long after the event has passed. These "exiled" parts are pushed away from conscious awareness because their pain is too overwhelming. Yet, they don't disappear; instead, they linger beneath the surface, ready to resurface at the most unexpected moments. For example, when your spouse makes a thoughtless remark, it can feel like a spark igniting a hidden flame. In an instant, you might be swept back to childhood feelings of unworthiness, reacting not just to the present comment but to echoes of past hurt. In that moment, the sting of a few careless words pulls us into a deeper pain, reminding us of times when we felt small and overlooked.

Unresolved trauma can manifest in multitude of ways—such as constant anxiety, bouts of depression (emotional dysregulation), physical symptoms, self-sabotage, or a persistent sense of imbalance. One might even result to seemingly positive coping mechanisms which we'll cover in a later chapter. These aren't just passing emotions; they're deep wounds that shape our perspective on the world and influence how we connect with others. In parenting, these wounded parts can lead us to react in ways that protect ourselves rather than respond to our children's needs. A mother burdened by feelings of inadequacy might become overly critical or distant, not from lack of love for her child but in an attempt to shield herself from more pain. This creates a cycle where unresolved trauma quietly disrupts the ability to nurture and connect.

It's important to identify these parts as it helps us understand the roots of these traumas. And it is also important to approach this process with compassion rather than judgment. Recognizing the existence of these parts and the burdens they carry allows us to engage with them gently and with curiosity. This compassionate approach helps us to start the journey toward healing. In IFS, this involves supporting these parts in releasing their pain, which frees us to interact with the world, and our children, from a place of peace rather than pain.

Engaging in this healing work is essential as it lays the groundwork for our own freedom. It's not merely about alleviating personal suffering; it's about breaking the cycle of trauma to prevent it from affecting future generations.

By approaching this inner journey with compassion we can cultivate a more balanced and resilient version of ourselves, one capable of offering our children the emotional support they need to thrive. Healing unresolved trauma with kindness and patience is a powerful act of love, creating ripples that extend beyond our own lives and positively impact the hearts of those who follow.

When we take our final breath, the healing we've embraced continues to echo forward. The legacy we leave behind isn't in the business empires but in how courageously we chose to face our pain, to heal our wounds, and to offer this gift of freedom to the next generations. Every small step we take toward healing ensures that our children, and their children, will carry fewer burdens, experience deeper love, and walk their own path with greater strength and resilience and without the shadows of trauma.

The Connection between Trauma and Impulsive Decisions in Mothers

"Self-control is an umbrella construct that bridges concepts and measurements from different disciplines (e.g., impulsivity, conscientiousness, self-regulation, delay of gratification, inattention-hyperactivity, executive function, willpower, intertemporal choice)" (Moffitt et al., 2011). Impulse control refers to the ability to pause before reacting, allowing individuals to think critically before making decisions or taking action. For instance, when you spot a pair of shoes you want, impulse control encourages you to evaluate whether the purchase is necessary or fits your budget, rather than succumbing to the immediate urge to buy them. But trauma can significantly disrupt this ability, making it more challenging to regulate emotions and control impulses, often leading to hasty decisions or emotional outbursts.

Understanding how trauma affects impulse control and decision-making is crucial. Maybe this has not crossed your mind in the past, but hear me out.

Unaddressed trauma can trap the brain in "survival mode," where immediate threats overshadow emotional balance and the ability to see beyond the now, much less envision a much hopeful future and long-term planning. In this state, the brain remains on high alert, reacting impulsively to perceived dangers. This heightened state complicates calm and collected thinking and decision-making aligned with long-term goals.

Trauma also greatly influences specific parts of the brain, particularly those developed as protective mechanisms during difficult experiences. For instance, childhood events such as physical abuse, emotional neglect, or witnessing domestic violence can contribute to the formation of "manager" parts, as described in Internal Family Systems (IFS) theory. These manager parts are driven by emotions like fear, anxiety, and guilt, focusing on maintaining control and avoiding vulnerability.

"Gail & Jake"

Consider Gail, an eight-year-old with a worn teddy bear hugged tightly in her arms. Sitting alone on the edge of the couch, she glances at the front door, waiting for her mother's familiar footsteps. Each tick of the clock feels like a reminder of her growing worry. What if she doesn't come back?

To distract herself, she begins to line up her toys on the floor, arranging them with a seriousness that belies her age. Each toy is placed carefully, one by one, as if creating a little army against the chaos that threatens her world.

When the door finally creaks open, Gail jumps up, a bright smile on her face, even though her heart races with anxiety. "I've been waiting!" she calls out, trying to sound cheerful while her eyes scan her mother's face for any sign of reassurance.

In that moment it's clear: Gail's need to control her environment comes from a deep-seated fear of being let down. Rather than showing her vulnerability, she builds a wall around herself, hoping to feel safe in a world that sometimes feels unpredictable.

Similarly, a child who faces constant criticism or emotional invalidation may develop a manager part driven by the fear of feeling inadequate. This part pushes them to make quick decisions or act impulsively, trying to avoid those deeper feelings of worthlessness or shame.

Take Jake, for example. At just nine years old, he often felt like he was tiptoeing around his home, where his parents' sharp words could pierce through the quiet. Every mistake seemed to open the door to criticism, leaving him anxious and unsure of himself.

In class, when the teacher asked questions, Jake would blurt out answers before he had a chance to think. It was like a reflex—if he spoke quickly, he hoped to dodge the awkward silence that followed his mistakes. Each hasty answer was his way of protecting himself, a small shield against the feelings he didn't want to face.

Whenever uncertainty crept in, whether it was a surprise quiz or a group project, Jake felt a familiar knot of anxiety tighten in his stomach. To manage that anxiety he often jumped to conclusions, making snap decisions just to regain a sense of control. But deep down, he knew this wasn't the best way to handle things.

In these moments, Jake's manager part kicked in, fueled by the fear of not being good enough. Instead of allowing himself to feel vulnerable, he kept himself busy, thinking that if he just moved fast enough, he could escape the shame lurking beneath the surface.

As adults, both Gail and Jake carry pieces of their childhood struggles with them, often without even realizing it, and these experiences shape their lives and relationships in significant ways.

Gail, now in her thirties, finds herself sitting in a conference room with her colleagues. The clock ticks loudly on the wall and as the meeting drags on she feels a familiar knot of anxiety tighten in her stomach. When discussions turn to who will take on new projects, she jumps in without thinking, volunteering for more than she can handle. *What if they think I can't keep up?* The fear of being seen as inadequate pushes her to overcommit, trying to avoid any hint of rejection.

At home, this tendency to control surfaces in her relationships too. Gail constantly double-checks plans with friends, worried that any sign of disinterest means they'll abandon her. When her partner is late, her mind races with worries, imagining the worst scenarios. Deep down, she knows her overactive imagination stems from her past, but letting go of that control feels like stepping into the unknown.

Jake, on the other hand, is now a software developer in his late twenties, staring at his computer screen filled with lines of code. As deadlines loom, he rushes to finish projects, convinced that speed will earn him his boss's approval. *What if I mess this up?* The fear of not measuring up pushes him to make impulsive choices, opting for quick fixes instead of taking the time to find the best solution.

In social situations, Jake's impulsivity shines through. He often interrupts friends mid-sentence, eager to jump in with a comment or joke. He worries that if he doesn't keep the energy high, he'll be forgotten or overlooked. Even as laughter fills the room, there's a part of him that feels distant, his thoughts swirling with self-doubt. He craves deeper connections but struggles to let his guard down enough to truly connect with others.

Both Gail and Jake navigate their adult lives with a sense of urgency, trying to manage the fears and anxieties that linger from their childhoods. Their inner manager parts push them to control their surroundings and avoid vulnerability, making it tough to embrace the uncertainty that life brings. While they recognize these patterns, they also know that the journey toward healing and self-acceptance is vital, even if it feels daunting at times.

As you reflect on Gail's and Jake's stories, do you see echoes of their experiences in your own life? Perhaps you find yourself overcommitting like Gail, driven by a fear of rejection; or maybe you relate to Jake's impulsivity and need for approval. Recognizing these patterns is a step toward understanding yourself better and finding a path toward healing. What steps can you take to embrace your own vulnerabilities and break free from the fears that hold you back?

By understanding these manager parts and their emotional triggers through Internal Family Systems (IFS) mothers—and really anyone—can start to gain better control over their impulses. When we take the time to look deeper, we often find that these parts are driven by a desire to protect us, even if their methods aren't always helpful. They're trying to keep us safe, usually from the pain of old wounds we might not even realize we're carrying.

When we begin addressing the underlying wounds that activate these protective strategies, we open the door to making more thoughtful, balanced decisions in our daily lives. Instead of reacting from a place of stress or fear we find the space to pause, reflect, and respond in ways that serve us better. This shift not only improves emotional regulation but also enhances our overall well-being, allowing us to show up more fully for ourselves and those we love. We unlock a deeper capacity to experience joy, compassion, and connection that makes our interactions richer and our relationships more fulfilling.

Imagine the ripple effect of this transformation as we grow more attuned to our inner world; we naturally become more grounded, patient, and present. Our children benefit from witnessing our healing, learning through our example how to process their own emotions with gentleness and understanding. We become a safe harbor for them, just as we are learning to become one for ourselves. The beauty of this work is that it's never too late to begin (take it from me). Every step toward self-awareness is a victory and each time we bring kindness to the parts of us that feel hurt or scared we heal a little more each time. When we create a foundation of emotional resilience that not only transforms our lives, we ultimately empower future generations to live with more love, more empathy, and courageous strength.

What Is the Survival Brain?

You may have heard of the "survival brain," the instinctive part of our minds that reacts automatically to perceived threats. This concept, rooted in our evolutionary biology, illustrates how our brains are wired for protection. Understanding its role can be an important step in personal development. Goleman (1995), a psychologist and science journalist known for his work on emotional intelligence, emphasizes that emotional awareness is essential for developing the skills needed to manage our emotions effectively. By learning to move beyond these automatic responses you can enhance your emotional regulation and significantly improve your overall well-being. For those just beginning this journey, remember that every step toward self-awareness is a meaningful accomplishment.

Learning to recognize and shift away from survival-driven reactions can introduce a variety of benefits that greatly enhance your daily experience. Improved emotional regulation empowers you to handle challenging situations—whether navigating unexpected changes to your carefully arranged schedule or engaging in difficult conversations—while remaining calm and collected. This newfound clarity enables you to manage daily stressors more effectively, such as juggling work deadlines with personal commitments or addressing minor setbacks with a focused mindset. You will likely notice significant improvements in your relationships; for instance, you may find yourself more engaged during family dinners, cherishing quality moments with your children, and participating in deeper, more meaningful conversations with friends. Just as resisting the impulse to buy another pair of shoes can enhance financial decision-making, cultivating greater emotional balance fosters clearer thinking in your financial choices and a more focused approach to achieving personal goals.

Let's See How the Survival Brain Works:

1. **The Brain's Alarm System**: At the core of the survival brain is the brain's alarm system, primarily driven by the amygdala, a small almond-shaped cluster of nuclei in the temporal lobe. The amygdala is responsible for processing emotions and detecting threats. When it senses danger, it triggers a cascade of physiological responses to prepare the body to either fight, flee, freeze or fawn.

2. **Activation of the Stress Response**: When you encounter a perceived threat, the amygdala sends signals to the hypothalamus, which then activates the adrenal glands. These glands release stress hormones, such as cortisol and adrenaline, into the bloodstream. These hormones prepare your body for immediate action by increasing your heart rate, sharpening your senses, and directing blood flow to vital organs and muscles.

3. **Focus on Immediate Threats**: This stress response, while crucial for dealing with immediate danger, can become problematic when it's triggered by less immediate, everyday stressors. When trauma is unresolved, your brain may remain in a state of heightened alertness,

constantly scanning for potential dangers. This can make you more sensitive to stress and less able to manage everyday challenges effectively.

4. **Impact on Daily Life**: When your brain is stuck in survival mode, even minor incidents can feel overwhelming. Your responses may become more intense and emotionally charged because your brain interprets them as threats. This heightened state of alertness can lead to difficulties in maintaining emotional balance and making thoughtful decisions. You might react impulsively or struggle to calm down, even in situations where a more measured response would be appropriate.

5. **Hypervigilance and Emotional Regulation**: When in survival mode, you might experience hypervigilance—a persistent state of heightened alertness and anxiety. According to an article in *Psychology Today*, hypervigilance is often characterized by an overwhelming sense of being constantly on guard, which can significantly disrupt your ability to regulate emotions (Sullivan, 2022). This ongoing state of vigilance can lead to considerable challenges; it complicates stress management and makes it increasingly difficult to maintain a sense of calm. The stress associated with hypervigilance also takes a toll on your physical health, contributing to fatigue, irritability, and chronic tension. Furthermore, it can strain relationships as you may struggle to connect emotionally with others or respond to their needs effectively. Living in a state of constant alertness can exhaust you and create barriers to meaningful, supportive interactions with those around you.

Hormones, Stress, and Motherhood

Motherhood comes with its own set of emotional and physical demands and when trauma is part of the picture, it makes managing stress more challenging. Hormones play a huge role in how our bodies handle stress, but if you've been through trauma, your stress response can stay heightened, throwing your hormones out of balance. This can lead to things like mood swings, feeling constantly drained, or even physical health issues like weight gain or fertility problems. It doesn't just affect your health—its impacts trail to those around you. Understanding how trauma, stress, and hormones are all connected can help us better manage our health and our relationships with our families.

A. Chronic Stress and Hormonal Dysregulation

1. Understanding the Stress Response:

- **HPA Axis Activation**: The **HPA axis** (hypothalamic-pituitary-adrenal axis) is a system in our body that helps us respond to stress. When we experience stress, the hypothalamus in the brain releases a hormone called CRH. This triggers the pituitary gland to release another hormone called ACTH, which tells the adrenal glands to produce cortisol. Cortisol helps the body manage stress by providing energy and regulating important functions. However, when someone experiences trauma, this system can become overactive, leading to persistently high levels of cortisol. This chronic stress can result in various health problems. In short, the HPA axis plays a crucial role in how our body handles stress and trauma.
- **Impact of Chronic Stress**: Prolonged elevated cortisol levels can disrupt the balance of other hormones, such as insulin and sex hormones (e.g., estrogen, progesterone, testosterone). This can lead to conditions such as:
    - **Insulin Resistance**: Cells become less responsive to insulin, leading to elevated blood sugar levels and potentially type 2 diabetes.

- o **Reproductive Hormonal Imbalances**: Stress can affect the menstrual cycle, leading to irregular periods, fertility issues, and symptoms of premenstrual syndrome (PMS).

2. Cycle of Stress and Health Issues:

- **Feedback Loop**: Chronic stress leads to hormonal imbalances, which can cause further stress and anxiety. For example, insulin resistance can lead to weight gain, which may trigger negative body image and self-esteem issues that further perpetuate stress.
- **Behavioral Responses**: Elevated cortisol can lead to cravings for unhealthy foods (high in sugar and fat) as a coping mechanism, creating a cycle of poor dietary choices and further exacerbating hormonal imbalances.

B. Mental Health Impact

1. Connection to Anxiety and Depression:

- **Neurotransmitter Regulation**: Hormonal imbalances can affect neurotransmitters like serotonin and dopamine, which are crucial for mood regulation. This can increase susceptibility to anxiety and depression, particularly for mothers who may already be experiencing heightened stress from parenting.
- **Trauma Triggers**: Past trauma can manifest in parenting situations (e.g., feeling overwhelmed by a child's needs), triggering stress responses that exacerbate mental health issues.

2. Impact on Parenting:

- **Emotional Availability**: Mental health challenges can affect a mother's emotional availability toward her children, impacting

attachment and the mother-child bond. This can perpetuate a cycle where the child's needs are not met, leading to stress for both the mother and child.
- **Generational Trauma**: Unresolved trauma can be passed down through generations as children may internalize their mother's stress and emotional dysregulation, potentially leading to their own trauma responses.

C. Physical Health Outcomes

Long-Term Health Consequences:

- **Metabolic Disorders:** Chronic stress and hormonal dysregulation can lead to obesity, metabolic syndrome, and type 2 diabetes, all of which are prevalent among individuals with a history of trauma. These conditions often arise from the body's altered responses to stress, including increased appetite and cravings for unhealthy foods.
- **Cardiovascular Diseases:** There is a significant link between elevated cortisol levels and increased blood pressure and heart rate, heightening the risk of cardiovascular diseases. This is particularly concerning for mothers, who often juggle multiple responsibilities and stressors, leading to heightened vulnerability.
- **Autoimmune Diseases/Disorders:** The chronic activation of the stress response can trigger or exacerbate autoimmune diseases, such as rheumatoid arthritis, lupus, and multiple sclerosis. Stress-induced inflammation may alter immune responses, leading to the body mistakenly attacking its tissues. This can manifest in various symptoms, including fatigue, joint pain, and skin issues, complicating the health challenges mothers face as they manage both their own health and family responsibilities.

Physical Symptoms of Stress:

- **Somatic Symptoms:** Trauma can manifest physically through symptoms such as chronic pain, digestive issues, and fatigue, affecting a mother's ability to care for herself and her children. These somatic symptoms often arise as the body expresses unresolved emotional distress, leading to a cycle of pain and fatigue.
- **Immune System Suppression:** Prolonged stress can suppress immune function, making mothers more susceptible to infections and illnesses, which further impacts their health and well-being. This suppression is particularly concerning for those with autoimmune disorders as stress can exacerbate symptoms and increase flare-ups, leaving mothers feeling overwhelmed and vulnerable.

The Persistent Effects of 9/11: Collective Trauma

Many of us might recall the morning of September 11, 2001. I had just picked up some textbooks and was strolling across campus when I stumbled upon the cafeteria. The normal student bustle was gone. Instead, it was unusually silent. People flocked around with their eyes fixed on the wall monitors. Something was wrong. Everyone's expressions were of surprise and horror as if time had stood still. I paused, trying to figure out what was going on, but everything changed right then.

That day did more than simply shock us in the moment. For many, the impacts of 9/11 have persisted, woven into the fabric of our lives in ways we may not even be aware of. This day still haunts and hurts those who were there and millions who watched helplessly from afar 23 years later.

The Long-Term Consequences

Trauma, especially on such a massive scale, doesn't simply fade with time. Many individuals who witnessed or experienced the events of 9/11 still grapple with symptoms of post-traumatic stress disorder (PTSD), anxiety, and depression. The fear and uncertainty that permeated the weeks, months, and even years following the attacks still resonate today. Some have never fully processed the trauma, leaving deep emotional scars that persist in their daily lives.

But the impact of trauma isn't just emotional—it has profound physical effects as well. Chronic stress, particularly when left unresolved, can wreak havoc on the body. Stress from trauma can disrupt the normal functioning of the body's systems, particularly the immune and endocrine systems, leading to long-term health consequences. This can manifest in increased susceptibility to illnesses, chronic pain, digestive problems, and even autoimmune diseases.

Both survivors and those affected remotely have experienced a wide range of health issues due to the lingering stress from 9/11. Many individuals have reported persistent symptoms of stress-related illnesses, such as insomnia, heart disease, and even cancer. The burden of this trauma can weigh heavily on families, with parents often struggling to manage their own health while caring for their children. This is especially true for mothers, who may feel the weight of maintaining normalcy for their families while silently dealing with the emotional and physical toll of their own unresolved trauma.

The event also triggered a new wave of collective trauma, where individuals across the country and beyond absorbed the fear, uncertainty, and grief that rippled through society. Many were left feeling vulnerable in a way they hadn't before. The pervasive sense of loss and danger that 9/11 introduced continues to influence our collective psyche, creating stressors that have impacted people's health in subtle and sometimes unrecognized ways.

The Lasting Effects of Trauma and Stress

The emotional and physical toll of trauma, whether from an event like 9/11 or from personal, unresolved experiences, builds up over time. What many don't realize is that when trauma isn't fully processed, it doesn't just disappear—it gets stored in the body. As Dr. Gabor Maté states, "Trauma is not what happens to you but what happens inside you as a result of what happens to you" (Maté, 2003). That constant state of stress triggers a cascade of responses, from hormonal imbalances to immune system dysfunction.

Living in survival mode for too long can cause the body to misfire, leading to a range of health problems that may seem unconnected to the original trauma. This is where many individuals, especially mothers, find themselves years or even decades later: battling health issues that don't always have a clear explanation. The connection between chronic stress, trauma, and long-term health conditions—like autoimmune disorders—becomes clearer when we understand how stress keeps the body in a state of constant alert, eventually wearing it down.

For some, these health issues surface as fatigue or chronic pain; for others, they manifest as more serious conditions like autoimmune diseases, where the body begins to attack its own tissues. The body's inability to return to a state of balance after ongoing trauma or stress can explain why so many people today are struggling with unexplained health issues.

And this is where we see the hidden yet powerful link between trauma, stress, and the onset of autoimmune disorders.

Autoimmune Diseases/Disorders

Chronic stress can significantly impact immune system function, potentially triggering or exacerbating various autoimmune diseases. Here's a more extensive list of common autoimmune disorders that can affect individuals, especially mothers, under prolonged stress:

1. Rheumatoid Arthritis (RA):

- **Description:** An inflammatory disorder that primarily affects joints, causing pain, swelling, and stiffness. It can lead to joint damage over time.
- **Connection to Stress:** Stress can increase inflammation in the body, worsening symptoms and potentially triggering flare-ups.

2. Lupus (Systemic Lupus Erythematosus):

- **Description:** A complex autoimmune disease that can affect multiple organs, including the skin, kidneys, and heart, causing a range of symptoms from fatigue to joint pain and skin rashes.
- **Connection to Stress:** Stress may exacerbate lupus symptoms and increase the frequency of flares.

3. Multiple Sclerosis (MS):

- **Description:** A disease where the immune system attacks the protective sheath (myelin) covering nerve fibers, leading to communication problems between the brain and the rest of the body. Symptoms can include fatigue, mobility issues, and cognitive changes.
- **Connection to Stress:** Stress can contribute to MS flare-ups, potentially accelerating the progression of the disease.

4. Hashimoto's Thyroiditis:

- **Description:** An autoimmune disorder where the immune system attacks the thyroid gland, leading to hypothyroidism, characterized by fatigue, weight gain, and depression.

- **Connection to Stress:** Chronic stress can lead to hormonal imbalances that may trigger or worsen Hashimoto's symptoms.

5. Graves' Disease:

- **Description:** An autoimmune disorder that causes hyperthyroidism, characterized by symptoms such as weight loss, anxiety, and rapid heartbeat.
- **Connection to Stress:** High stress levels can influence thyroid hormone production and worsen symptoms.

6. Psoriasis and Psoriatic Arthritis:

- **Description:** Psoriasis is a chronic skin condition characterized by red, scaly patches, while psoriatic arthritis affects the joints, causing pain and stiffness.
- **Connection to Stress:** Stress can trigger flare-ups of psoriasis and worsen the joint pain associated with psoriatic arthritis.

7. Type 1 Diabetes:

- **Description:** An autoimmune condition where the immune system attacks insulin-producing cells in the pancreas, leading to high blood sugar levels.
- **Connection to Stress:** Stress can complicate diabetes management, making it more difficult to maintain stable blood glucose levels.

8. Celiac Disease:

- **Description:** An autoimmune disorder where ingestion of gluten leads to damage in the small intestine, resulting in gastrointestinal issues and malabsorption of nutrients.

- **Connection to Stress:** Stress may worsen symptoms and lead to non-compliance with dietary restrictions.

9. Sjogren's Syndrome:

- **Description:** An autoimmune disorder that primarily affects the glands that produce moisture, leading to dry mouth and dry eyes, and can also cause joint pain and fatigue.
- **Connection to Stress:** Stress may aggravate symptoms and affect overall quality of life.

10. Myasthenia Gravis:

- **Description:** A neuromuscular disorder characterized by weakness and rapid fatigue of voluntary muscles, caused by communication breakdown between nerves and muscles.
- **Connection to Stress:** Stress can worsen muscle fatigue and exacerbate the condition.

11. Scleroderma:

- **Description:** A group of autoimmune diseases that cause the skin and connective tissues to become thick and hardened. It can also affect internal organs.
- **Connection to Stress:** Stress may exacerbate symptoms and influence disease progression.

12. Vasculitis:

- **Description:** Inflammation of blood vessels that can restrict blood flow to various organs and tissues, leading to serious complications.
- **Connection to Stress:** Chronic stress can trigger flares in various types of vasculitis.

These autoimmune diseases illustrate the wide range of conditions that can be influenced by chronic stress. Mothers, who often experience unique stressors related to caregiving and family responsibilities, may find their autoimmune symptoms intensified, leading to a cycle of health challenges that can affect both their physical and mental well-being. Understanding this connection is vital for effective management and support.

Trauma and Maternal Instincts

Trauma affects maternal instincts by prioritizing immediate safety over emotional connection. This isn't a reflection of your abilities as a mother but rather your brain's attempt to protect you from perceived threats. When in survival mode, bonding and nurturing might feel distant or overwhelming.

Imagine your brain is always scanning for danger, overshadowing natural instincts to bond and care. This constant vigilance can lead to moments of warmth but also periods of withdrawal or irritability. Understanding this struggle can help you be kinder to yourself, recognizing that these challenges stem from past experiences, not a lack of love or capability.

"One Moment at a Time"

You press your forehead against the kitchen window, fingers lightly tracing the droplets that cling to the surface. Outside, the sounds of children laughing and leaves rustling fill the air, but inside a heavy silence wraps around you like a thick blanket.

On the couch, your teenage daughter is sprawled out, headphones in place, completely absorbed in her phone. You feel the urge to reach out, to bridge the gap between you, but something keeps you rooted in place. An invisible weight settles in your chest and your mind races, scanning for threats that exist only in your imagination.

Remember the pure joy of cheering her on during those childhood milestones? When she first rode her bike or performed in that school play? Those moments felt like sunshine, radiating warmth and love. But now that warmth seems buried beneath layers of anxiety and past trauma, making it hard to feel close.

As she laughs at something on her screen, it tugs at your heart. You crave that connection, but vulnerability feels daunting. The clock ticks softly in the background, a reminder that you're still here, still a parent, even amidst the struggle.

Taking a deep breath, you push through the heaviness. You walk over to the couch, heart racing. "Hey, want to watch something together?" you ask, trying to keep your tone casual.

She glances up, a smile breaking through her concentration. In that moment, something shifts inside you. Love is still there, waiting for you to reach out. It won't be perfect, but you know you can take it one moment at a time, embracing the small steps toward connection.

Navigating Motherhood in Survival Mode

Navigating motherhood while in survival mode is a challenging experience. When you're constantly focused on immediate threats, it can overshadow the nurturing aspects of parenting, heightening anxiety and making it difficult to bond with your child. Recognizing these survival responses is the first step toward healing. By becoming aware of your nervous system's protective patterns, you can create moments of mindfulness and self-compassion even amidst the chaos. This awareness not only helps you identify your triggers but also empowers you to respond with intention rather than react out of habit, allowing you to process past trauma and rediscover the joys of parenting.

Have you ever felt like everyday stressors are hitting you harder than they should? If you're constantly in survival mode, remember that your brain's primary job is to keep you safe. It's so focused on protecting you from perceived threats that it has little capacity left for experiencing positive emotions or nurturing your natural instincts. Unresolved trauma can heighten this state of alertness, making even minor challenges feel overwhelming and affecting your impulse control and decision-making. This heightened vigilance doesn't just impact how you respond; it can also make it harder to trust your maternal instincts and connect with your children the way you'd like to. Understand this isn't about self-blame; it's about recognizing why you react the way you do.

By acknowledging how trauma impacts both your responses and your ability to connect with your children you can begin to understand yourself better, begin to heal and foster a more nurturing environment at home. This awareness helps you build a more stable, supportive, and connected family, allowing for deeper, more meaningful relationships with your children.

The Impact of Past Trauma on Mom's Mental Health

We're slowly realizing that the struggles we face as mothers aren't just about present-day challenges but reverberations of our pasts. Many of us may not recognize that our current difficulties—like feelings of inadequacy or challenges connecting with our children—often stem from a lack of positive modeled behavior during childhood. As Dr. Bessel van der Kolk (2014) notes, "The past is never dead. It's not even past," highlighting how experiences of trauma and challenging relationships can leave lasting impacts that shape our perceptions and interactions in adulthood. When we understand these roots, we can address our struggles more effectively and begin to foster healthier connections with our own children. Research indicates that unresolved emotional wounds from childhood, such as abuse or neglect, can resurface during critical life transitions like pregnancy, childbirth, and early motherhood. These unresolved traumas often manifest as anxiety, which, if left unaddressed, may escalate into more severe mental health conditions such as chronic depression or PTSD (BMC Psychiatry, 2024).

Birth Trauma and Retraumatization

When a woman becomes pregnant, the focus often shifts entirely to the baby. Throughout pregnancy, medical appointments tend to focus on the baby's development and standard health questions like smoking, drinking, and family medical histories. However, what is often overlooked is the emotional well-being of the mother and any past traumas that could resurface. In my experience, I was never asked about my emotional history or informed about the possibility of retraumatization during childbirth. Only after doing my own research did I realize I wasn't alone. There is such a thing as **birth trauma** and **retraumatization**, though it's rarely discussed in maternal care.

This lack of awareness had a profound impact on me, especially after the births of my daughters. I experienced postpartum depression and intense feelings of rage. At the time, I didn't understand why I felt so overwhelmed or why my emotions were so difficult to control. I often wondered if my past traumas were somehow connected to these feelings.

The Birth Experience: A Complex Emotional Terrain

Childbirth is a time of vulnerability for all mothers, but for those with a history of childhood trauma it can be especially challenging. The intense physical sensations, loss of control, and emotional demands of labor can trigger unresolved trauma. Ford and Courtois (2020) explain that "experiences involving loss of control, physical invasion, or intense emotions can often trigger a re-experiencing of trauma for survivors of childhood abuse" (p. 45). This was true for me. I often felt powerless during childbirth, which resurfaced old feelings of fear and helplessness from my past.

Birth Trauma: What It Means and How It Happens

Birth trauma refers not only to physical complications but also to the emotional distress that can occur during or after childbirth. Even when the birth process itself is medically smooth, mothers with trauma histories can still experience it as deeply disempowering. Beck et al. (2013) found that "feeling disempowered during birth, either through lack of communication or control, is a common factor in traumatic birth experiences, especially for women with a history of trauma" (p. 24).

For me, this was a major factor. After giving birth, I struggled with postpartum depression and, even more unexpectedly, postpartum rage. I felt this uncontrollable anger surge up in me at times and it was terrifying. I had no idea that this could be connected to my past traumas. In retrospect, it makes sense: feelings of helplessness and powerlessness during childbirth can easily mirror past experiences of trauma, intensifying the emotional aftermath.

Retraumatization: When Birth Echoes the Past

Retraumatization happens when current experiences trigger emotions or sensations tied to past trauma. For mothers like me, with childhood trauma, the physical and emotional intensity of birth can act as a powerful trigger. Reynolds (2013) points out that, "mothers who experienced childhood trauma are at a higher risk of dissociation during childbirth, as the physical pain and loss of control may mirror traumatic memories of helplessness" (p. 78). This is exactly how I felt—not just during the birth but in the months that followed. My body and mind seemed to react to the birth in ways that I couldn't fully understand or control, leading to overwhelming emotions like rage and sadness.

The postpartum period was extremely difficult. I struggled to make sense of why I felt so angry and hopeless at times. I now realize that birth, while a joyful event, can also bring buried trauma to the surface. The physical vulnerability, loss of control, and the sheer intensity of childbirth likely stirred up unresolved emotions from my past. As Van der Kolk (2014) famously explains, "The body keeps the score" (p. 36), meaning that traumatic memories often reside in the body, resurfacing when the body experiences similar sensations or stress.

Healing and Moving Forward: Recognizing and Addressing Trauma

Understanding that my past trauma may have played a role in my postpartum depression and that rage has been an important part of my healing I've come to learn that recognizing the potential for retraumatization during childbirth is key to preparing emotionally for the birth experience and for postpartum recovery. Trauma-informed care, as Goldsmith et al. (2020) advocate, "prioritizes the mother's sense of control and choice, fostering a safer emotional and physical environment during labor" (p. 121). If I had known about this approach earlier, I might have felt more prepared and supported.

For mothers with similar trauma histories, taking steps to safeguard emotional well-being during pregnancy and postpartum is crucial:

- **Trauma-informed care**: Working with healthcare providers who understand trauma and can respect the mother's autonomy and emotional safety.
- **Emotional support**: Having a trusted support person or doula present to help ground the mother emotionally and advocate for her needs.
- **Therapy and preparation**: Engaging with a trauma-informed professional, like a therapist or a coach, before birth to develop coping strategies and identify potential triggers.

Knowing what I know now, I realize that my past trauma did affect my postpartum experience. Understanding this connection has helped me to move forward in understanding myself even better as I begin to heal and I hope that sharing my story can help others feel less alone.

Studies have shown that women with a history of childhood trauma are at a higher risk of developing postpartum depression and anxiety as these vulnerable periods can trigger memories of past traumas (BMC Psychiatry, 2024). Specifically, postpartum PTSD can develop from traumatic childbirth experiences, especially in women with pre-existing trauma. Symptoms can range from flashbacks and hypervigilance to difficulty bonding with their children, all of which can profoundly affect a mother's mental health and family life. Recognizing the role of past trauma is crucial as early mental health interventions during pregnancy or postpartum periods can help mitigate these long-term risks.

Without awareness, recognition and intervention these unresolved issues can disrupt our emotional balance and limit our ability to be the mothers we strive to be. How might it feel to finally move past these burdens once we recognize and address them? Imagine the freedom and clarity we could experience if we weren't bogged down by these hidden influences but instead embraced the opportunity for healing and growth.

How Unresolved Trauma Affects Parenting Styles

Unresolved trauma can subtly shape our parenting style and influence how we react to our children. For instance, some individuals may become overly protective, where the drive to keep their children safe becomes overly controlling, potentially restricting their children's freedom and personal growth. According to Lange, Callinan, and Smith (2019), parents with a history of trauma may respond to their children's behaviors with increased anxiety, leading to exaggerated reactions. For example, a parent who experienced trauma related to safety might overreact to their child's minor accidents or mistakes, such as a scraped knee or a spilled drink. In such cases, the parent might say, "I can't believe you're always so careless! You never listen to me!" or "How many times do I have to tell you to be more careful?"

This overprotectiveness, driven by the parent's own fears and unresolved issues, can lead to reactions that include frustration or anger, even blaming the child for the mishap. Behind the scenes, this can significantly impact the child's perception of themselves. When children receive messages like these, they may begin to see themselves as clumsy, inadequate, or unworthy of trust. They might internalize the blame and start believing that their mistakes make them a disappointment or that they must always be perfect to avoid criticism. This rising feeling of not being good enough can hurt their self-esteem and make it harder for them to explore, take healthy risks, and develop independence.

On the other hand, some people may emotionally retreat to avoid dealing with past hurts. This emotional detachment can also negatively impact our children's sense of security and connection. For example, a parent with unresolved trauma might become emotionally unavailable during challenging times, spending long hours in isolation, mindlessly scrolling through social media or playing games on their phone to escape. In these moments, they may show little interest in their child's needs, saying things like, "Can't you see I'm too tired to deal with this?" or "I can't handle this right now—figure it out on your own." This withdrawal increases the disconnection even further and makes the child feel invisible.

As a result, the child may feel abandoned or rejected, interpreting the parent's withdrawal as a signal that they are not valued or that their emotional needs are inconvenient. Lack of involvement might cause the child to feel alienated and unsupported, which would affect their sense of self-worth, security and trust. Over time, the child may struggle with feelings of insecurity and develop a belief that emotional support is unreliable or that they are undeserving of attention and care.

Recognizing how our trauma influences parenting is key to breaking cycles of emotional pain and disconnection. By becoming aware of these patterns we can begin to heal ourselves and, in turn, improve our relationships with our children. Addressing unresolved trauma helps us build stronger, more secure bonds, creating a home where love, understanding, and emotional growth thrive. This shift not only helps our children feel confident and emotionally secure but also better prepares them to face life's challenges. Ultimately, we set them up for healthier relationships and a future rooted in emotional well-being.

Passing Down Trauma through Generations

When my mother was pregnant with me, our lives were shattered by a devastating fire that destroyed our home. To make matters worse, just months later, the house across the street also burned. This traumatic event led to my premature birth and, as I reflect on its impact, I can't help but wonder about the far-reaching effects of such early trauma on my own life.

Generational trauma is a concept that reveals how the wounds of one generation can echo through multiple layers of family history. As Kira et al. (2016) explain, intergenerational trauma involves the passing down of trauma's effects from one generation to the next, often leading to emotional and behavioral challenges. While my mother's trauma was immediate and profound, I question how deeply these effects have permeated my own family. The pain and stress she endured could ripple through generations, influencing behaviors and emotional responses in ways that might not stop with her.

Even if I were to uncover the deep-seated traumas my ancestors faced, what real benefit does it offer my children and their future if I don't take meaningful action to break this cycle today? It's not just about understanding the past; it's about transforming our present to ensure that our children grow up free from the shadows of unresolved pain. If we do not address and heal these patterns now, the cycle of trauma will persist, affecting generations to come.

Interactive Exercise: Self-Assessment Tool

At the end of this chapter, you'll find a self-assessment tool designed to help you identify gaps that might be influencing your parenting. Take a few minutes to fill it out thoughtfully. This quiz is here to support your journey of self-awareness, a crucial first step toward becoming the next improved version of yourself.

Self-awareness involves recognizing how your past experiences shape your thoughts, emotions, and behaviors today. It's about shining a light on the hidden parts of you, those patterns and triggers that may have been influencing your actions without you even realizing it.

Understanding these aspects of ourselves is powerful because it allows us to make more conscious choices in how we respond to life's challenges, especially in our role as a parent. Remember, this isn't about assigning blame or feeling guilty—it's about empowering yourself with knowledge. We often don't know what we don't know and that's perfectly normal. The process of uncovering these hidden influences can be challenging, so be gentle with yourself. Approach this with curiosity and compassion, knowing that every insight brings you one step closer to healing, growth, and, ultimately, a more fulfilling and connected life.

> "When you know better, do better"
> Maya Angelou

For me, enduring significant traumas from a young age built an emotional wall so solid that it kept some of those painful memories buried for decades. I often questioned my sanity, feeling as if I was "crazy" because I couldn't connect the dots between my past pain and my current emotional responses. This sense of being fundamentally flawed became even more glaring when I became a mother. It hit me hard. I would lash out over the smallest things—a spilled cup of milk here, a messy room there. For crying out loud, they were just babies, innocent and full of love. Even after I snapped, they'd come running back, arms open for a hug or ready to play, as if they'd completely forgotten my harsh words. They didn't know the depth of my struggle; they just wanted to connect.

It's excruciating to think that I was meant to be their safe haven yet I was the one causing the storm. What I didn't realize then was that their tiny hearts and minds were absorbing and storing these moments as core memories, shaping their sense of self and future in ways I couldn't fully grasp at the time. Reflecting on how I yelled at them over what now seems so trivial breaks my heart. After those outbursts, I would retreat into myself, overwhelmed by guilt and self-doubt, feeling unworthy of the incredible gift of motherhood. Those moments left me wrestling with my ability to be the nurturing, patient mother I so desperately wanted to be. I should have known better because this was the same painful beginning that had shaped my own life. The echoes of those early wounds followed me throughout my life, leaving a lasting mark on who I became.

Finding Ways to Cope and Get Help

Navigating motherhood while dealing with unresolved trauma can be overwhelming, but there are ways to lighten this load. Alongside gaining awareness, a crucial step is recognizing that the trauma exists. Naming it gives us power, transforming vague feelings of distress into something tangible that we can address. One effective approach is developing emotional granularity—being able to pinpoint and describe your emotions in detail. Instead of simply feeling "bad," you might identify specific emotions like "frustration," "sadness," or "anxiety." This clarity helps you understand what you're experiencing and how to manage it.

I'm sure you've experienced the calming power of deep breathing. For me, it's been a true lifesaver. It's simple and quick—just a few minutes of deep breaths can bring a sense of calm and clarity even in the midst of chaos. Another supportive tool is journaling, including what's known as a "brain dump," where you freely write down everything on your mind. This can help clear mental clutter and create a safe space to work through your feelings without judgment. Embracing these practices is a gentle way to help manage your stressors and support your emotional well-being.

Let's not forget the importance of self-compassion. Healing isn't something we can rush—it's a journey, not a race. So give yourself compassion and be patient along the way. Celebrate the small wins because each one helps build resilience and a more positive mindset. If you've never felt validated, this practice is even more powerful—it helps you find that validation within yourself. As you do, it strengthens your well-being and gives you the emotional foundation to support your children.

Dealing with unresolved trauma, especially as a mom, is tough. But recognizing the path you've taken and affirming your experiences is a big part of healing. It can feel lonely, but embracing your emotions for what they are brings a sense of freedom and peace. Remember, you are not alone.

As you move forward, you'll learn healthier ways to manage stress and triggers, which helps create more nurturing, positive relationships with your children. Taking care of yourself—whether that's through creativity, staying active, or carving out time just for you—plays such an important role in your overall health and healing. These little acts of self-care add up, contributing to your long-term well-being and even longevity. So, be kind to yourself—you deserve it.

QUIZ

Self-Assessment Quiz: Identifying Unresolved Trauma in Your Relationships

Instructions: For each statement, select the response that best describes how often you experience or relate to the situation. Be honest with yourself—this is a tool for self-awareness and growth.

Scale:
Never (0 points)
Rarely (1 point)
Sometimes (2 points)
Often (3 points)
Always (4 points)

1. I find myself reacting more strongly to situations than they seem to warrant.

2. Certain behaviors or situations trigger intense emotions, such as anger, fear, or sadness, in my relationships.

3. I often feel like I'm reliving parts of my own childhood when I interact with others, including my children.

4. I struggle with feelings of anger, guilt, shame, or inadequacy in my relationships.

5. I avoid certain conversations or topics with others because they remind me of painful memories.

6. I notice that I impose unrealistic expectations on myself or others, similar to those placed on me when I was young.

7. When someone I care about is upset, I find it difficult to remain calm and often feel overwhelmed.

8. I catch myself saying things to others that were said to me in hurtful ways by my own parents, caregivers, or significant people in my life.

9. I have difficulty trusting others, fearing they will let me down or hurt me.

10. I find it challenging to connect emotionally with others, often feeling distant or disconnected.

11. I struggle with setting healthy boundaries in my relationships, either being too lenient or overly strict.

12. I often feel like I need to protect myself or others from the world in ways that go beyond normal concern.

13. I experience flashbacks or vivid memories of my own childhood during stressful interactions with others.

14. I feel a deep fear of making the same mistakes in my relationships that my parents or caregivers made with me.

15. I notice a pattern of overreacting to small issues in my relationships then feeling regret or confusion afterward.

Scoring:

0–15: You likely have a healthy relationship with your past, though it's always helpful to stay mindful of your emotions and reactions.

16–30: You may have some unresolved issues from your past that occasionally influence your relationships. Consider exploring these areas further to enhance your connections with others.

31–45: It's likely that unresolved trauma from your past is impacting your relationships more than you realize. It might be beneficial to seek additional support or resources to address these areas.

46–60: Your past experiences are significantly influencing your relationships. This may be affecting both your well-being and the well-being of those around you. Consider seeking professional guidance to work through these challenges.

Reflection:

After completing the quiz, take some time to reflect on your responses. Which areas stood out to you? Were there any surprises? Understanding these patterns is the first step towards making positive changes in your relationships and your overall emotional health. Remember, self-awareness is a powerful tool for growth and this quiz is just the beginning of your journey.

Next Steps:

Grab your journal and jot down your thoughts after taking the quiz. Did anything surprise you? Like realizing that your reaction to your child's epic meltdown might be connected to your own childhood drama over, say, getting grounded for not cleaning your room? How does this new insight change the way you view your reactions and behaviors? Reflect on how these past experiences might be shaping your current responses and interactions with your kids. We'll dig deeper into this in the next chapters, exploring how to address and heal from these past wounds.

"Laundry Aversion"

There were only two bedrooms in our apartment and I had to share one with my baby brother and the "nanny." When I was nine years old, I woke up to an awful, overpowering smell that instantly made my heart race. This scent was unlike anything I had ever encountered; it was deeply unsettling and sent chills down my spine. My senses surged as I became acutely aware of something amiss. I would never forget that night, a vivid memory etched in my mind, marking the beginning of a distressing journey into fear and awareness.

The fear that had consumed me drowned out the familiar scents of fresh rain and the faint hint of laundry detergent from the nook outside our window. It wasn't just the scents themselves that frightened me; it was the eerie, suffocating feeling of an unknown presence right next to me. I lay completely still, pretending to be asleep, hoping that if I didn't move, I could somehow avoid any danger. That night, I was filled with paralyzing fear and a sense of vulnerability that stayed with me long after the stench had faded.

This sensation wasn't new to me; it was a familiar, troubling feeling I had experienced in my toddler years. I had grown up with this sense of dread, but it wasn't until I was of age that it became particularly vivid, frightening, and pure horrendous. I remember it all. I remember everything with the clarity of a noonday.

As I grew older, the smell of rain would often bring me to a place of profound despair, almost feeling like a cloud of depression would settle over me. I couldn't understand why a natural, soothing scent could affect me so deeply, but it was a constant reminder of that fear and vulnerability from my childhood.

For years, I couldn't figure out why doing laundry felt like such a chore. Over time, I began to notice a pattern of triggers—seemingly random and unconnected—that left me both puzzled and frustrated. Eventually, I recognized the deep connection between these aversions and emotional wounds from my childhood. The scents of rain and laundry detergent had become powerful triggers, pulling me back to that unspeakable night, moments of utter fear and perplexing memories.

Understanding that these reactions stemmed from past traumas helped me realize that unresolved emotions from early experiences, not a lack of willpower, were holding me back. It's important to know that many of us unknowingly carry these burdens and there's no shame in that. By gently acknowledging and exploring these emotional triggers we begin a compassionate journey of healing. With time, this process fosters greater self-awareness and empowers us to break free from the hold it has on us.

CHAPTER 4

The Invisible Saboteurs

Understanding Triggers:

Imagine you're hosting a family dinner, trying to balance lively conversations and the clinking of dishes. Suddenly, your sister-in-law makes a casual remark about your parenting choices and it feels like a lightning bolt just struck you. Your face heats up and your chest tightens with a wave of defensiveness and hurt. A warm, connecting evening has transformed into a battlefield, revealing old wounds and unresolved emotions.

Then your child bursts into the room, beaming with pride as they show you their latest artwork. But instead of sharing in their excitement, you're overwhelmed by a cloud of anxiety and self-doubt. What should be a joyful moment now feels like a spotlight on your insecurities, amplifying every concern you have about your parenting. The artwork, meant to be a celebration of their creativity, instead mirrors your deepest worries, making it difficult to enjoy the precious moment with them. As you struggle with these emotions your child senses your agitation and reacts harshly, turning their excitement into frustration and deepening the emotional turmoil of the moment.

These situations act as concealed emotional minefields dispersed throughout your life, triggering intense reactions that may appear abrupt and overpowering. To navigate these triggers more effectively it's helpful to understand them through the lens of Internal Family Systems (IFS) therapy.

The Psychological Impact of Triggers on Moms:

Triggers can greatly influence our emotional state, be it from past experiences, societal pressures, or the everyday demands of motherhood. They often bring up unresolved feelings or fears, and when they hit, it can feel like a tsunami crashing over us, making even the smallest tasks seem impossible. It's like the trigger opens the floodgates to emotions we haven't had a chance to process and suddenly we're struggling to keep everything together. As noted by the National Alliance on Mental Illness (NAMI), "Triggers can range from memories of past experiences to external stimuli that cause emotional reactions" (NAMI, n.d.).

The constant pressure to remain calm, gentle, and caring can intensify mothers' emotional stress. When we encounter a trigger and fall short of these expectations, it often leads to guilt or feelings of inadequacy. The internal narrative can become harsh, filled with self-criticism for not being able to maintain the image of the "perfect mother." It creates a cycle where the guilt only makes things harder and daily challenges feel even more overwhelming.

For example, something as simple as a comment from a family member or stress about your child's upcoming project can stir up a lot of emotions. These triggers often tap into deeper worries, like whether we're doing enough for our kids or meeting societal expectations for motherhood. This can lead to a mix of emotions that leave us feeling drained and doubtful about our parenting skills.

The emotional chaos from triggers can make us question our ability to stay composed, especially when we feel like we need to "hold it all together." Instead of feeling supported, we feel isolated, as if we're alone in our struggles.

The ideal of being the perfect mother—always patient, always nurturing—can make us feel even more inadequate when reality doesn't match up. This sense of isolation can make it harder to seek help or express how we're feeling, which only adds to the emotional burden.

It's important to remember that triggers aren't a sign of weakness or failure. They're just a part of the complex experience of motherhood and our emotional landscape. By acknowledging and dealing with these emotional responses we can start to find healthier ways to cope, allowing ourselves to be imperfect without self-judgment. Shifting our perspective can help lighten some of the pressure, making it easier to approach motherhood with more compassion for ourselves and a clearer understanding that perfection is neither necessary nor realistic.

How IFS Explains Triggers:

In IFS therapy, we recognize that our psyche is composed of various "parts," each holding specific emotions, memories, and beliefs. These parts often originate from past experiences and traumas. When a trigger occurs—such as a seemingly innocuous comment from a family member or a moment of personal reflection—it can activate these parts, bringing their stored emotional responses to the forefront.

For instance, the remark from your sister-in-law may activate a part of you that holds unresolved pain or insecurity from past experiences, such as feeling judged or criticized. This part might react defensively, causing you to feel hurt and threatened, even if the comment wasn't intended to be hurtful. Similarly, when you're faced with your child's artwork, a different part of you that holds fears or doubts about your parenting might be triggered, making you feel anxious and self-critical.

Recognizing and Managing Triggers:

Getting to know your personal triggers involves introspection and self-awareness. Start by paying attention to your emotional responses in different situations. When do you feel overwhelmed or irritable? What's happening right before those feelings hit? Often, triggers are tied to past experiences or unresolved issues.

1. Identifying the Parts: To manage triggers effectively, start by identifying which parts of you are being activated. For example, if a remark from your sister-in-law triggers defensiveness, it may be coming from a part of you that feels undervalued or criticized. Similarly, if you experience anxiety in response to your child's artwork, it might stem from a part that worries about your parenting competence.

2. Understanding the Reactions: Recognize that these reactions are often driven by specific parts holding past traumas or unmet needs. Your intense emotions may seem disproportionate to the immediate situation because they are reflections of deeper, unresolved issues rather than the current trigger alone.

3. Observing and Documenting Triggers: Keep a journal to document moments of intense emotions like anger, anxiety, or sadness. Record the situations and your immediate reactions. Over time, you'll spot recurring themes and patterns that can reveal underlying triggers. Pay attention to physical reactions, such as a racing heart or tense muscles, which can signal underlying triggers.

4. Reflecting on Past Experiences: Consider past experiences or core beliefs that might be influencing your current responses. Reflecting on these can help you understand your triggers better and how they relate to your emotional reactions.

5. Practicing Mindfulness: Stay aware of your emotional responses by practicing mindfulness. Observe your reactions in real-time and ask yourself what specifically triggered your response. This awareness can help you manage your reactions more effectively.

6. Seeking Feedback: Share your experiences with a trusted friend or close family members. Their observations can offer valuable insights into your triggers and help you gain a deeper understanding of your emotional responses. Approach these conversations with an open mind, recognizing that they might bring up strong emotions or uncomfortable truths. Defensive reactions are natural, but they can also be opportunities for growth and deeper understanding. **Disclaimer:** Choose supportive and trustworthy individuals for feedback. If discussions become too overwhelming, consider stepping back or seeking professional guidance.

7. Using Self-Help Resources: Read books and articles and use online tools to gain a deeper understanding of emotional triggers and self-awareness. Self-help resources can provide additional strategies and insights for managing triggers effectively.

8. Managing Triggers: Once you identify the different parts within you and understand their origins, you can utilize techniques such as self-compassion, mindful awareness, and *unblending* which involves separating from the activated part to respond to triggers with greater calmness and clarity. As highlighted in *Psychology Today*, Woolley (n.d.) notes that unblending is the practice of recognizing when you're triggered and distancing yourself from that activated part. This allows your true self to regain control, helping you acknowledge the feelings of those triggered parts without letting them dominate your reactions. By doing this you can navigate situations with greater balance and mindfulness.

In those moments, you might ask yourself, "What part of me is feeling this way and how can I create space to respond more thoughtfully?"

Growing Through the Process:

Understanding our triggers is like learning to drive a car. When we identify what sets us off, it's like recognizing different road signs and hazards along the way. This awareness helps us navigate our emotions more smoothly, knowing when to slow down, speed up, or steer in a different direction.

Adding mindfulness to this process is like using a GPS system. Mindfulness helps us stay present and observe our thoughts and feelings without judgment, allowing us to spot potential obstacles early and create a pause between what happens and how we react. This pause gives us the chance to choose a better suited thoughtful response rather than reacting on impulse. Not only does this help us handle difficult moments, but it also encourages us to address issues in a more mindful and balanced way, supporting our overall emotional well-being.

Emotional Check-In

Before we dive into how to handle these triggers, let's take a moment to check in with ourselves. Take a deep breath and simply notice how you're feeling right now. It's perfectly okay to feel a bit frazzled or unsure as you begin to uncover what sets you off.

We're fortunate to live in a time when mental health matters and conversations around it are more prevalent. Our parents and their parents didn't always have the tools or understanding we have today to navigate trauma and emotional responses. This space is here for you to explore your feelings without judgment. Think of it as peeling back the layers of an onion—

sometimes it's messy and can even make you cry, but it's all part of getting to know yourself better.

Finally, maybe we can be the generation that breaks this cycle. Let's take the insights we gain and create a healthier narrative for ourselves and those who come after us.

Now, reflect on the last time you had a strong emotional reaction. What was happening in that moment? What emotions came up for you? This reflection can be incredibly helpful in pinpointing the root of those intense feelings. Remember, this journey isn't about self-criticism; it's about understanding and growth.

Common Triggers Moms Experience

Feeling Overwhelmed: Juggling the endless demands of parenting and household tasks can leave you feeling utterly exhausted and stressed. It's like being stuck on a treadmill that never stops, constantly trying to keep up but never quite catching a break. This sense of being overwhelmed is often cited in discussions within parenting forums and support groups.

Comparing Ourselves: Social media can intensify feelings of inadequacy. Seeing others 'seemingly perfect lives can make you feel like you're falling short. This comparison can stir up feelings of guilt and self-doubt. In a zero-sum mindset, we often view self-worth as a limited resource—if someone else is thriving it feels like our own value diminishes. Remember, social media is essentially a highlight reel, not the whole story.

Lack of Support: Many moms struggle with feeling like they're carrying the weight of everything alone. Whether it's a lack of support from a partner or family or feelings of isolation, these situations can be emotionally draining. This lack of support is a frequent topic of discussion in online parenting communities.

Child's Behavior: Public outbursts or challenging behaviors from children can trigger feelings of embarrassment and frustration. These reactions often stem from personal insecurities or stress.

Personal Past Trauma: Situations that echo past trauma, such as conflicts or stressors that remind a mother of unresolved issues from her own childhood, can provoke strong emotional reactions. Recognizing this trigger can be crucial in addressing underlying emotional needs.

You're doing important work by facing these triggers head-on. It might feel challenging, but remember you're not alone in this process. We're all here, working through these emotions together. Embrace this opportunity to learn more about yourself and to strengthen your emotional resilience. You've got the strength and courage to uncover and address these triggers and I'm here to support you every step of the way.

Next Steps:

Let's turn this into action. Take some time to write down the things that trigger you. What are the common patterns? How do these triggers make you feel? Use this list to create a plan for addressing and managing these triggers. We'll build on this in the coming chapters to develop coping strategies and tools for handling these emotional responses effectively.

Identifying your triggers reflections:

1. What Happened?
Describe the situation or behavior that triggered you. For example, did a particular action from your child set you off? Note down the specifics.

2. How Did You Feel?
Record your emotional response to the trigger. Were you frustrated, angry, overwhelmed, or something else?

3. What Might This Trigger Be Related To?

Reflect on whether this trigger reminds you of something from your past. Does it connect to a past experience or a recurring pattern in your life?

Review and Reflection

1. Look for Common Themes:

Review your completed worksheet and identify any recurring patterns or themes. What common threads link these triggers to your personal history or past experiences?

2. Understanding the Connection:

How do these triggers relate to your past? Use this insight to understand the deeper connections between your emotional responses and past experiences.

3. Create an Action Plan:

Based on your reflections, start developing strategies for managing and mitigating these triggers. Note down practical steps you can take to handle these emotional responses more effectively.

"The Buy-In to Belonging"

When I was in elementary school, everything felt like it was falling apart. My father had returned from working in the Middle East, but my mother had left again to chase new opportunities. Even though he provided for me financially, he was always working and rarely around. Money couldn't fill the emptiness left by his absence but it sure bought me some semblance of belonging.

My situation felt worse such that he disregarded the atrocity done to me by one of his own relatives. I felt deeply betrayed; my trust and boundaries had been completely shattered. In a desperate attempt to feel connected and valued, I started using the money he gave me to treat my friends. Whether it was buying snacks after school or paying for their roller skating, I hoped that by spending money on them they'd like me more and I'd finally feel like I belonged somewhere. I even used the money intended for my tuition to splurge on clothes, hoping that material things might fill the void and make me feel better. It was my way of trying to fix the hurt, even though I didn't fully understand what was wrong.

On top of everything, my school performance suffered terribly. My concentration was so poor that keeping up with lessons became nearly impossible. How could I focus on school when I was constantly overwhelmed by fear and my anxiety being on overdrive? The stress of my personal life made learning feel like an insurmountable challenge and I felt stuck in a cycle of failure and frustration.

As I moved into adolescence, I continued using these coping strategies to manage my stress and confusion. I became obsessed with trying to be perfect, achieving as much as possible, thinking that if I excelled in everything I'd finally feel good about myself and find a place where I truly belonged. This constant drive for perfection was exhausting and, despite my efforts, it never seemed to be enough.

In 2021, during the height of my depression and at my lowest point, I eagerly joined a mom group on Instagram, longing for connection and support. However, when I was kicked out for failing to adhere to their rules, it deepened my pain. What I had hoped would be a source of acceptance became yet another experience of rejection. In retrospect, though, that experience was a blessing in disguise; it forced me to confront the depths of my agony.

My need for perfectionism and desperation for validation stemmed from a deep-seated fear of rejection and feelings of inadequacy. I craved acceptance, wanting to be liked and valued, so I worked tirelessly to meet others' expectations, hoping to fill an imaginary hole and shield myself from further hurt.

This relentless pursuit of approval led me to seek validation from others, often at my own expense. I became adept at molding myself to fit what I thought others wanted, all in an attempt to secure a sense of belonging and worth. It took me a long time to realize that this need for validation and perfection was merely a façade to mask the deep pain and confusion I felt. True healing required me to face and address the underlying hurt I was trying so desperately to avoid.

CHAPTER 5

You're Not Okay

Introduction to Coping Mechanisms

Coping mechanisms are the strategies we rely on to manage stress and navigate life's challenges. These mechanisms become a crutch to maintain some sense of control and stability, especially those dealing with unresolved traumas. It's completely understandable that you might lean on these tactics to get through tough times.

However, it's important to recognize that not all coping strategies are equally effective or beneficial. Sometimes, what might seem like a positive approach on the surface can be masking deeper emotional issues and may even end up being counterproductive. This is not a reflection of failure but rather a common experience shared by many.

By exploring these coping mechanisms through the lens of Internal Family Systems (IFS) we can begin to understand how they often originate from parts of ourselves that are trying their best to protect us from past hurts that have yet to be addressed. These parts may have developed their strategies out of a real need to shield us from emotional damage, even if those methods no longer serve us well.

Recognizing that some of your old coping strategies might now be holding you back is a big step and it shows real growth. These strategies once helped you manage tough times, but as you change and grow, they might no longer be the best fit. This doesn't mean your past approaches were wrong—it's just that you're evolving and need new tools to match where you are now.

Understanding this can be unnerving, but it's also a chance for meaningful change. We are moving from surviving to thriving. By facing these deeper emotional wounds and exploring new, healthier ways to cope, you are giving yourself the chance to build a more fulfilling life.

It's also helpful to remember that this journey doesn't have to be solitary. There are people and communities out there who understand what you're going through and can offer support and guidance. Taking these steps towards deeper self-understanding is a sign of real strength and commitment to your own well-being.

Common Positive-Seeming Coping Strategies

Overworking and Busyness

It might seem like keeping yourself busy is a sensible way to deal with stress and stay in charge. A lot of women get caught up with scheduling numerous activities for their kids or doing too many things at work and at home. Chronic busyness is a way many people distract themselves from uncomfortable, unpleasant, and painful emotions. The busyness, the action, the constant movement, and the over-commitment actually protect the person from being aware of their emotions (Verywell Mind, n.d.; Psychology Today, n.d.). That being said, this tactic is often used to draw attention away from underlying inner wounds, even though it can make the person look efficient and productive.

Georgia's Story

Georgia, a mother of three, found herself constantly juggling her children's extracurricular activities, her job, and household chores. Despite appearing highly organized and productive, she was struggling with feelings of inadequacy and fear of failure. She later realized through therapy that her relentless busyness was a way to avoid confronting her deep-seated fears of not being a good enough parent. According to her therapist, Georgia's overworking was driven by a part of her trying to protect her from these uncomfortable feelings.

Perfectionism and Achievement

The pursuit of perfection can seem like a positive coping strategy. Mothers who strive for an idealized version of parenting or success often engage in behaviors driven by a need for validation and control. This quest for perfection can serve as a coping mechanism, helping mothers manage stress and feelings of inadequacy. By striving for perfection they may believe they can better handle their anxiety and fears of not being good enough. However, according to Curran and Hill (2019), this relentless pursuit can lead to additional pressure and dissatisfaction, highlighting the complex and harmful nature of perfectionism in modern times.

Maria's Experience

Maria, who had always strived to be the perfect mother and professional, frequently found herself emotionally exhausted and never quite satisfied with her achievements. Her perfectionism stemmed from a part of her personality trying to shield her from feelings of inadequacy. She realized that her drive for perfection was tied to deep-seated fears of not measuring up and addressing these fears allowed her to develop a healthier approach to her goals.

Constant Self-Sacrifice

Putting other people's needs ahead of one's own is often seen as a noble and kind gesture. However, consistently prioritizing taking care of others over one's own needs may lead to emotional depletion and self-neglect.

Mila's Journey

Mila, a single mother, consistently put her children's needs ahead of her own, initially feeling noble for her selflessness. However, this led to resentment and emotional exhaustion over time. Her self-sacrifice was rooted in the belief that her worth depended on her ability to care for others, a pattern often developed in childhood when caregiving roles were assumed in response to unmet emotional needs.

Recognizing that self-care is essential for maintaining emotional health was crucial for Mila. By finding a balance between her needs and those of her family she began to overcome the exhausting cycle of self-sacrifice.

Dissociation through Creativity

Dissociation can sometimes be harnessed positively through creative outlets, allowing individuals to manage stress and unresolved trauma. For some, engaging in creative activities can provide a way to channel emotions and maintain focus while navigating challenging experiences.

Eliza's Story

Eliza, a novelist and mother of three, used her writing as a way to cope with past trauma. By immersing herself in her fictional stories she found emotional detachment helped her manage personal challenges and remain productive. Her novels received acclaim and her ability to channel her struggles into her work was widely admired. In therapy, Eliza learned that while writing offered a valuable escape, addressing her trauma directly was essential for complete emotional healing.

The Hidden Costs of These Strategies

Burnout and Exhaustion

The relentless pursuit of busyness or perfection can lead to physical and emotional exhaustion. Recognizing signs of burnout, such as fatigue and irritability, is crucial.

Emotional Suppression

Avoiding or suppressing emotions is another hidden danger. By focusing on external activities or achievements individuals may avoid confronting their emotional struggles, leading to unresolved issues.

Neglecting Self-Care

Self-care is a vital component of emotional and physical health. When prioritizing others 'needs, individuals may overlook essential self-care practices, resulting in decreased well-being.

Increased Anxiety and Stress

Engaging in seemingly positive coping mechanisms can create pressure to maintain a certain image or lifestyle. This pressure can lead to heightened anxiety and stress, particularly if expectations are not met.

Difficulty Setting Boundaries

The desire to please others can make it challenging to set healthy boundaries. This can result in overcommitting and feeling overwhelmed as individuals may struggle to say no.

Loss of Identity

Focusing solely on others can lead to a loss of self-identity. When mothers or caregivers prioritize the needs of others over their own, they may lose sight of their personal goals, interests, and values.

Resentment and Frustration

Constantly putting others first can lead to feelings of resentment. Individuals may become frustrated when their efforts go unrecognized or unappreciated, leading to emotional distress.

Isolation

The focus on maintaining a façade of strength or competence can result in social isolation. Individuals may withdraw from friendships and support systems, believing they need to handle everything on their own.

Physical Health Issues

Chronic stress and neglect of self-care can lead to physical health problems, such as headaches, digestive issues, and weakened immune function, affecting overall quality of life.

Impaired Relationships

While the intention may be to maintain harmony, people-pleasing behaviors can create imbalances in relationships. Others may become reliant on the individual for validation, leading to unhealthy dynamics.

Stunted Personal Growth

Overemphasis on fulfilling others 'expectations can stifle personal growth and exploration. Individuals may miss opportunities to develop new skills or pursue passions that would enrich their lives.

Cognitive Dissonance

The gap between personal feelings and external actions can lead to cognitive dissonance. Individuals may struggle internally when their actions do not align with their true feelings, creating additional stress.

Addressing the Root Causes

By exploring these coping mechanisms through Internal Family Systems (IFS) we can understand that parts of ourselves driving these strategies are often attempting to protect us from deeper pain. For instance, a part driving perfectionism may be shielding us from feelings of inadequacy. Understanding these protective parts allows for a compassionate approach to addressing the root causes of coping mechanisms. By acknowledging and working with these parts you can start shifting towards healthier, more balanced strategies that promote genuine healing and well-being.

Moreover, engaging in this type of self-exploration can lead to significant emotional growth and resilience. Individuals who participate in inner dialogues often experience greater emotional regulation and a reduction in anxiety symptoms. Additionally, understanding the motivations behind our behaviors fosters self-compassion, which is linked to improved mental health outcomes. By cultivating a deeper awareness of our internal landscape we not only pave the way for personal healing but also create a more nurturing environment for ourselves and those around us.

Practical Tips and Interactive Exercises

To begin working with your protective parts and shifting towards healthier coping strategies, follow these steps:

1. Identify Your Coping Behaviors: Notice when you engage in coping strategies such as overworking, perfectionism, or constant self-sacrifice. Pay attention to the situations and emotions that trigger these behaviors.

2. Pause and Reflect: When you recognize a coping behavior, pause and ask yourself, "What is this part of me trying to protect me from?" This reflection helps you understand the underlying fears or feelings that are driving your behavior.

3. Acknowledge and Validate: Gently acknowledge the feelings or fears that this part is trying to shield you from. This step is crucial for building self-compassion and understanding the true source of your stress or anxiety.

4. Seek Support: Integrate self-care practices into your routine and consider seeking professional help if needed. This support can assist in addressing the underlying issues and finding healthier ways to cope.

Interactive Exercise: Identifying Your Coping Mechanisms

Reflecting on personal experiences with coping strategies can provide valuable insights into their effectiveness and impact. Take some time to evaluate your coping mechanisms with the following questions:

What are coping strategies and how can they vary?
Consider examples of coping strategies you've encountered, such as problem-

solving, seeking social support, or practicing mindfulness. Which of these resonate with you?

Why is it important to reflect on my coping strategies?
Think about times when you felt overwhelmed or stressed. How did your coping strategies help or hinder your situation?

What coping strategies do I rely on most often?
Make a list of the methods you use to manage stress and challenges. Do you notice a pattern, like being constantly busy or putting others' needs ahead of your own?

How do these strategies make me feel emotionally and physically?
Reflect on a recent situation where you used a coping strategy. What were your emotional and physical reactions afterward? Did you feel more relaxed, drained, or indifferent?

Are there patterns of behavior that might be masking deeper issues?
Identify any recurring behaviors you exhibit during stressful times. Do you find yourself avoiding certain feelings or situations? How might these behaviors relate to deeper emotional struggles?

How can I determine if my coping strategies are effective?
Think about specific outcomes you want from your coping strategies. Are they helping you feel better? Do they improve your mood or help you manage stress effectively?

What should I do if I find my coping strategies are ineffective?
Consider what changes you might make. Are there new strategies you'd be willing to try or could you seek support from friends or professionals?

How can I develop new coping strategies?
Explore resources like books, workshops, or counseling that could help you

learn new techniques. What strategies appeal to you and how could you incorporate them into your life?

Is it normal to struggle with coping strategies?
Reflect on your experiences and those of others around you. Have you seen or heard stories about people facing similar struggles? How does that make you feel about your own challenges?

Action Plan for Change

Develop a personalized guide to implement healthier changes and manage stress more effectively. Follow these steps to create your action plan:

1. **Outline Specific Steps**: Define actionable steps to integrate mindfulness practices, establish boundaries, and seek support. For example, allocate specific times each week for activities like yoga or journaling, set clear limits on after-work emails to protect personal time, and research local support groups or therapists to find the right fit for your needs.

2. **Set Realistic Goals**: Break down your goals into achievable steps. For instance, start with a five-minute daily meditation practice, gradually increasing to 15 minutes as you grow more comfortable, or aim to read one chapter of a self-help book each week to build resilience and insight.

3. **Review and Adjust**: Regularly assess your coping strategies to gauge their effectiveness. Schedule monthly check-ins to reflect on your progress, discuss any challenges you faced, and make necessary adjustments to your plan based on your experiences and changing circumstances.

Remember, acknowledging and working with your coping mechanisms is a courageous and important step towards healing. It's completely normal to have protective parts of you that have been trying their best to keep you safe, even if their methods have become unhelpful.

Be gentle with yourself as you navigate this journey. Change takes time and rarely follows a straight path, so it's completely okay to experience setbacks along the way. What truly matters is your willingness to approach these challenges with understanding and self-compassion. Remember, you are not alone—many mothers face similar struggles and seeking support is an act of courage and strength. Every small step you take toward self-awareness and healing brings you closer to a more balanced and fulfilling life and your commitment to improving your coping strategies will have a lasting impact on your well-being.

The Balance of Acknowledgment: It's Okay to Not Be Okay, But...

In recent years, the phrase "It's okay to not be okay" has become a mainstream mantra in conversations about mental health. While I wholeheartedly support the sentiment behind it—recognizing and validating our feelings is crucial for emotional well-being—it's also important to unpack the potential negative connotations that can arise from this statement.

On one hand, acknowledging that it's okay to not be okay allows individuals to embrace their struggles without fear of judgment. It creates space for vulnerability and opens the door for authentic conversations about mental health challenges. This acknowledgment can be liberating, empowering those who may feel pressured to present a façade of perfection or normalcy. It reminds us that everyone has moments of difficulty, pain, and uncertainty.

However, there is a risk that this perspective can inadvertently promote a victim mindset, where individuals find a sense of power in their struggles.

Subconsciously, some may derive comfort from identifying as a victim as it can provide a justification for inaction and a means to elicit sympathy from others. I used to often say that I was the way I was because of what happened to me, using my past experiences as a lens through which to view my current self. This perspective, while initially comforting, ultimately kept me from recognizing my own agency and capacity for change.

While validating feelings is essential, this mindset can create a cycle where individuals cling to their pain, believing that their struggles define them and that they have little control over their circumstances. Consistently accepting that it's okay to be in a state of struggle can lead to stagnation. If we linger too long in this acknowledgment without actively seeking paths to healing and improvement we may become trapped in a cycle of despair, feeling powerless to effect change in our lives.

Furthermore, the phrase can sometimes downplay the importance of taking steps toward recovery. Acknowledging our struggles should ideally be a catalyst for action—a first step toward seeking help, making changes, and fostering resilience. Brené Brown emphasizes this idea beautifully: "Our job is not to deny the story but to defy the ending—to rise strong, recognize our story, and rumble with the truth until we get to a place where we think, Yes. This is what happened. And I will choose how the story ends" (Brown, 2015). This encourages readers to acknowledge their pain while taking proactive steps toward healing and redefining their narratives. It's essential to balance this validation of our current feelings with the understanding that while it's okay to not be okay, it's equally important to strive for a better state of being.

In my own journey, I learned that recognizing and accepting my pain was just the beginning. It was the willingness to confront that pain, to actively seek healing, and to engage with supportive communities that truly set me on a path toward recovery. Thus, while I embrace the message that it's okay to not be okay, I also advocate for the importance of moving beyond that acknowledgment to foster growth, resilience, and a commitment to personal well-being.

"Pile of Dirty Dishes"

When I had my fifth child, I faced postpartum challenges that were far beyond anything I had imagined. Despite having been through this before, the difficulties I encountered with my youngest were raw and overwhelming. It felt as if the universe had decided it was time for me to confront the deepest parts of my unresolved trauma.

An intense wave of exhaustion and emotional chaos quickly overshadowed the joy of welcoming a new baby into the world. It became clear that my childhood trauma wasn't just a distant memory; it was ingrained in me and being a parent made it all come rushing back.

No amount of preparation or therapy could have truly prepared me for this. The physical demands of caring for a newborn were draining, but it was the emotional toll that truly exposed my unmet needs and unresolved issues. My children, in their pure, innocent way, were reflecting back to me the very wounds I had tried to bury. They didn't just show me my vulnerabilities—they revealed where I needed healing the most.

One night stands out clearly. My baby was only about three months old and, after a long night of nursing, I went into the kitchen to find a pile of dirty dishes. Suddenly, I was overwhelmed with a rage I couldn't control. I started throwing dishes and smashing them. It felt like all my hidden pain exploded at once and I was caught in a storm of anger. It was as if my inner child, who had been hurt and neglected, was breaking through my adult self. The outburst was both shocking and heartbreaking, a raw display of the deep pain I had been carrying inside.

I had always thought I was handling things well, but the challenges of a newborn forced me to face my old wounds. The constant demands and sleepless nights made it clear that I couldn't hide from the deep-seated issues from my childhood: feelings of self-doubt, inadequacy, and a fear of never being enough.

When my baby cried, it felt like a painful reminder of the neglect and unmet needs from my own past. My frustration wasn't just about the baby's cries—it was a powerful echo of the pain I had kept buried for so long. The hurt and ignored inner child within me was crying out, demanding the attention and love I hadn't given myself.

This realization was eye-opening. I understood that the love and care I was giving to my baby were also what I needed to give to myself. For the first time, I saw that to heal my old wounds I had to embrace and nurture those parts of me that had been crying out for help. This was a painful but crucial step in reprogramming the deep-seated beliefs that had been shaping my life.

What truly changed me was realizing that, while caring for my baby's innocence, I was also beginning to heal my own. As I tended to my baby with unconditional love I started to notice small but significant changes in myself. Taking care of someone so vulnerable helped me reconnect with my own lost innocence. Through this process of giving and receiving love I slowly started to heal.

Parenting wasn't just about raising kids—it became a journey of uncovering and healing parts of me that needed attention. As I nurtured their innocence I found a way to reconnect with my own. This experience changed how I saw myself, helping me face and shift deep-rooted beliefs that had shaped my life. Looking back, I realize the love we give our children has a way of consoling us too. By embracing our weaknesses and allowing parenting to transform us we can start to heal our deepest, most painful scars.

CHAPTER 6

Your Brain Isn't Your Bestie

Imagine waking up each day feeling empowered, where your thoughts and beliefs align perfectly with the life you envision. This transformation begins with reprogramming your subconscious mind—the quiet force behind your reality. Although it may feel like a close, lifelong companion, your subconscious mind is more like an old friend who influences your decisions without you even realizing it. Early experiences shaped this "friend," quietly forming patterns that guide your thoughts, feelings, and reactions to the world around you—even when you're not paying attention.

For those still dealing with the effects of past traumatic events, these ingrained responses can feel like an invisible wall, much like outdated software limiting performance. The positive news is that you have the power to reprogram these patterns and reshape your life. Think of neuroplasticity as the brain's built-in update system—an incredible capacity to rewrite old code by forming new neural connections. Just like software that isn't static and adapts with new updates, your brain continuously evolves based on your experiences and learning. You are always capable of creating a new version of yourself, optimized for growth and resilience.

Here is where Neuro-Linguistic Programming (NLP) can make a significant difference. NLP provides practical techniques for transforming thought patterns and emotional responses. By applying this method you can alter the internal maps that guide your reactions, effectively reprogramming your subconscious to support your goals and aspirations. Though not exhaustive, techniques such as reframing, anchoring, and visualization are tools that will help you shift from old, limiting beliefs to new, empowering ones.

Understanding the Subconscious Mind and Its Protective Role

As you may recall from the earlier chapters about Maslow's Hierarchy of Needs, the brain prioritizes safety and well-being as fundamental needs. From the moment of birth, your subconscious mind begins to develop, absorbing and shaping experiences up until around the age of seven. These formative years create a blueprint for how you respond to life's challenges. Your subconscious interprets early experiences through a protective lens, striving to ensure a sense of security. For instance, if a child experiences trauma or neglect, the subconscious may develop coping mechanisms that persist into adulthood. This could manifest in various ways, such as when a mother with unresolved childhood trauma feels overwhelmed by her child's tantrums as her subconscious reactivates old, unhealed wounds.

Many of us find ourselves stuck in repetitive behaviors and it can feel like we're on a hamster wheel—going through the motions but not really getting anywhere. Whether it's mindlessly scrolling on our phones instead of focusing on important tasks or reaching for comfort food during stressful moments, these habits can seem almost impossible to break.

But here's the good news: these behaviors are learned, not set in stone. For instance, if you tend to procrastinate when faced with a daunting project, that tendency likely developed over time, perhaps as a way to cope with anxiety. Understanding that these automatic responses are not permanent can be incredibly empowering. It means that, with some effort and mindfulness, you can start unlearning these patterns. Stay with me!

Imagine replacing that late-night snack with a relaxing tea or setting specific times for social media use instead of letting it take over your day. These small changes can lead to healthier habits that align more with your goals. Change might take time and patience, but the potential for growth is always within your reach.

Recognizing the outdated programs influencing your values and actions is the first step in initiating this transformation. Think back on how previous events shaped your present ideas and behavior. One useful method for revealing and organizing deep-seated ideas is journaling. Watch your emotional triggers; they expose underlying attitudes and unresolved trauma. By documenting these triggers and connecting them to limiting beliefs you can begin using NLP techniques to reframe and replace them with empowering, supportive beliefs.

Tools and Techniques for Reprogramming

1. CULTIVATING GRATITUDE

The rise of gratitude practices in recent years can be attributed to a mix of scientific research, growing awareness about mental health, and the power of modern media. Just about every day, it seems, we come across posts on TikTok or Instagram with hashtags like #grateful, where people share the small and big things they're thankful for. Studies show that gratitude can significantly enhance mental and emotional well-being. Despite any past experiences or limiting beliefs that might have shaped your perspective, incorporating gratitude into your life can help you:

A. Focus on the Positive (Gratitude Practice)

Actionable Steps:

- **Start small:** Each day, write down three things you're grateful for. They can be as simple as having a good cup of coffee or a conversation with a friend.
- **Set a reminder:** Use your phone or a journal app to set a daily notification to practice gratitude.
- **Track progress:** After a week, look back on your list. Noticing how the small positives add up can help reinforce the habit.

Why it works: Regularly identifying things to be thankful for trains your brain to look for positives, something that has been shown to improve mood and well-being over time.

B. Spark Curiosity (Cultivate Exploration)

Actionable Steps:

- **Ask one new question daily:** For example, "What can I learn from this situation?" or "What's something I've always wanted to explore more?" This builds a habit of curiosity.
- **Try a "new thing" challenge:** Each week, commit to trying something different (a new food, a new route home, or reading an article on a topic you don't know much about).
- **Set a curiosity goal:** Maybe it's reading one book a month or attending a free workshop. This adds structure to your curiosity practice.

Why it works: By consistently looking for novelty you're engaging the brain's reward system, which keeps you more engaged and excited about life.

C. Welcome Change (Growth Mindset)

Actionable Steps:

- **Reframe challenges:** The next time you face a tough situation, instead of asking, "Why is this happening to me?" ask, "What can I learn or gain from this experience?" It shifts your mindset toward growth.
- **Set small, adaptive goals:** When life changes, set specific goals that allow you to move forward. For example, if you've just started a new job, aim to meet one new colleague each day.
- **Reflect regularly:** Take time at the end of each week to note any changes you've faced and how you adapted. This reflection helps reinforce your resilience.

Why it works: Welcoming change and actively seeking out the lessons in it can make you more adaptable and resilient in future challenges.

Action Steps:

To start a gratitude practice it's beneficial to draw on the work of two influential figures in positive psychology: Dr. Robert Emmons and Dr. Martin Seligman. Dr. Emmons, a leading researcher on gratitude, has demonstrated that maintaining a gratitude journal—where individuals list things they are thankful for—can significantly enhance well-being and happiness. In his book *Thanks! How the New Science of Gratitude Can Make You Happier* Emmons (2007) discusses how gratitude practices can lead to increased positive emotions and life satisfaction.

Meanwhile, Dr. Martin Seligman, a pioneer in the field of positive psychology, introduced the "Three Good Things" exercise. This simple yet powerful practice involves noting three positive events or experiences from your day and reflecting on why they happened. In his book *Authentic Happiness: Using the New Positive Psychology to Realize Your Potential for Lasting Fulfillment* Seligman (2002) outlines how this exercise can enhance happiness and overall life satisfaction.

With these insights in mind you can begin your own gratitude practice by starting a Gratitude Journal. Each day, write down three things you are grateful for or try Seligman's "Three Good Things" exercise. Visualize these as vibrant, shiny objects in your "gratitude jar" and feel the warmth and lightness of each entry. This practice helps to counteract limiting beliefs and aligns with the proven benefits of embracing gratitude in your daily life.

Express Appreciation: Make it a habit to regularly acknowledge and thank others for their positive impact on your life. Martin Seligman emphasizes that expressing gratitude not only strengthens relationships but also boosts personal well-being. Picture their smiles and feel the warm, uplifting sensation of gratitude spreading through your chest. This simple act of appreciation can break through any past conditioning that might be holding you back, fostering a more open and positive mindset. For further reading, Seligman's book *Flourish* provides insights into how gratitude practices enhance happiness and life satisfaction.

2. UNDERSTANDING AFFIRMATIONS & REPROGRAMMING THE MIND

Affirmations are positive statements that can help shift your thinking and overcome negative beliefs. When used regularly, they have the potential to reprogram your subconscious mind and change how you view yourself. However, it's important to use them as part of a balanced approach to self-improvement. They're not a cure-all and shouldn't replace addressing deeper issues or emotions. Also, watch out for toxic positivity—where focusing on being positive can sometimes dismiss or invalidate real struggles. Affirmations should support your overall journey and not overshadow the importance of recognizing and working through all your feelings and seeking extra support when needed.

Why Do Affirmations Work?

Affirmations have become a vital part of my life, helping me gradually replace negative beliefs with positive ones. In *Psycho-Cybernetics*, Maxwell Maltz (1960) emphasizes that transforming our self-image through affirmations is key to achieving real personal growth. He shares stories from his work as a plastic surgeon, where he noticed that patients who changed their self-perceptions often experienced significant improvements in their quality of life, regardless of any physical changes they underwent.

Maltz describes the subconscious mind as a "servo mechanism," constantly working to help us achieve our goals based on how we see ourselves. By regularly affirming my worth and potential I've been able to program my subconscious to support these positive beliefs. This has created a kind of feedback loop in my life: As I nurture positive thoughts I find myself taking positive actions, which in turn has helped gradually boost my self-esteem and leads to greater success.

Through this practice I've discovered that regularly repeating affirmations strengthens the neural connections in my brain, or "wiring," which makes it easier to access positive thoughts over time. This frequent activation leads to the "firing" of these pathways, reinforcing positive thinking and allowing me to break free from long-standing negative patterns that once held me back. My mood and well-being improve with affirmations, which boost resilience and optimism. Inspired by Maltz's insights, I take time to vividly visualize my goals while I repeat my affirmations. This powerful combination has truly transformed my practice, resulting in meaningful changes in my behavior and self-perception.

Factors Influencing the Effectiveness of Self-Affirmation Interventions

Self-affirmation practices can offer significant mental health benefits, particularly for mothers navigating the complexities of parenthood and unresolved trauma. However, I want to address how mainstream affirmations have become, with many people touting their magical transformation stories. While these narratives can be inspiring it's important to remember that what works for one person may not work for another. It's essential to approach these techniques with realistic expectations. I don't want to leave you with false hope or promises that self-affirmation will be a one-size-fits-all solution. The effectiveness of these practices can vary widely based on individual circumstances. To better understand this variability, let's look at some research findings. Research indicates that factors such as personality traits, mental health status, and personal experiences can significantly influence how well these interventions work.

For instance, a study focusing on self-affirmation interventions for adults with psoriasis found that specific approaches—like those centered on body image—did not always outperform more general self-affirmation methods. This suggests that the type of affirmation may not be as critical as previously thought. Additionally, the study revealed that age and self-esteem can greatly influence outcomes. Mothers with higher self-esteem often find affirmations more effective while those grappling with trauma or mental health challenges might need more comprehensive strategies to see meaningful improvement.

Recognizing that you are not alone in overcoming these issues is critical. Many moms face comparable challenges and realizing your unique path is the first step toward healing. Tailoring self-affirmation activities to your needs can be quite powerful. In conclusion, consider reflecting on your strengths and values as this can serve as a foundation for crafting affirmations that resonate deeply with you.

Here are a few supportive strategies to enhance your affirmation practice:

- **Personalize Your Affirmations**: Create affirmations that speak directly to your experiences and feelings. For example, instead of a general affirmation like "I am strong," try something more specific like "I am strong enough to overcome my past and be the mother I want to be."
- **Practice Self-Compassion**: Remember that it's okay to have tough days. Be gentle with yourself and recognize that healing is a journey. Incorporating self-compassion into your affirmations can foster a more nurturing mindset.
- **Engage with a Support Network**: Share your affirmation journey with friends, family, or support groups. Surrounding yourself with those who uplift and encourage you can strengthen your resolve and help you stay motivated.
- **Reflect on Your Progress**: Take time to acknowledge the small victories in your journey. Reflecting on your growth can reinforce positive thinking and boost your self-esteem.

These insights remind us that affirmation practices should be flexible and tailored to each mother's unique circumstances. By embracing your individual journey and adapting self-affirmation techniques to suit your needs you can cultivate a deeper sense of empowerment and resilience. Remember, seeking support and understanding your own strengths are powerful steps toward creating a fulfilling life for yourself and your family. Together, we can continue to explore these strategies and enhance the way we approach self-affirmation in our everyday lives.

The Neuroscience Behind Self-Affirmation

Understanding how self-affirmation influences our brains can shed light on why these practices are so effective, especially for mothers navigating the complexities of parenthood and personal challenges. Research shows that self-affirmation activates specific areas in the brain associated with self-reflection and value assessment, which can lead to significant mental health benefits.

When individuals engage in self-affirmation—reflecting on their core values and what makes them feel worthy—they experience increased activity in key brain regions. For instance, the **medial prefrontal cortex (mPFC)** and **posterior cingulate cortex (PCC)** become more active, indicating that the individual is deeply engaging in self-reflective thinking. This heightened activity helps reinforce a positive self-image, making it easier for mothers to regain confidence, especially when faced with stress or feelings of inadequacy.

Think of the mPFC as your internal cheerleader. When you reflect on the things you value—like your ability to nurture your children or your commitment to your personal goals—this part of your brain lights up, reminding you of your strengths and capabilities. This can be especially empowering when you're feeling overwhelmed.

Moreover, self-affirmation activates the **ventral striatum** and the **ventral medial prefrontal cortex (vmPFC)**, areas linked to reward processing and value recognition. This means that thinking about one's values not only feels good but also makes these values seem more significant and motivating. For mothers who may often place their needs last this neural response can be a powerful reminder of their worth, encouraging them to prioritize self-care and positive change.

Imagine the ventral striatum as the part of your brain that responds to rewards, similar to how you feel when you indulge in a treat or receive praise. When you affirm your values, it triggers that same sense of satisfaction and motivation, pushing you to take steps that are good for you, like taking a break or asking for help when needed.

Real-World Impact on Behavior

The implications of this brain activity extend beyond just feeling good. The research indicates that when mothers engage in self-affirmation, they are more likely to adopt healthier behaviors, such as increasing physical activity. This is particularly important for those dealing with the pressures of motherhood and unresolved trauma as it provides a path toward greater emotional and physical well-being.

By understanding that these positive changes in brain activity can lead to actionable outcomes mothers can appreciate the tangible benefits of self-affirmation practices. Recognizing that their brains are responding positively to these affirmations can empower them to continue using these techniques, fostering resilience and promoting good mental health.

Neural Pathways

Do you like working out? Just like exercising your body strengthens your muscles, repeating affirmations can help strengthen your brain. When you consistently practice positive affirmations—those uplifting statements about you or your life—you're exercising your brain and creating new neural pathways.

This is where neuroplasticity comes into play. It's the brain's amazing ability to reorganize itself by forming new connections throughout our lives. By regularly practicing affirmations you encourage your brain to focus on positive thoughts, making it easier to access those uplifting feelings in the future.

So, just as lifting weights can build physical strength, repeating affirmations can enhance your mental resilience. Over time, this practice can lead to a more optimistic mindset, allowing you to handle challenges and setbacks with a positive attitude.

Mood and Well-Being

Research shows that affirmations can significantly boost mood and enhance overall well-being. Studies indicate that self-affirmation not only helps reduce stress but also improves performance by encouraging individuals to focus on their values and strengths. For example, a study published in *Social Cognitive and Affective Neuroscience* revealed that self-affirmation activates the brain's reward centers, leading to a more positive outlook. This relationship between self-affirmation and mood improvement highlights its potential benefits for mental health, making it a valuable practice for anyone looking to enhance their emotional state.

Self-affirmation and Stress

Self-affirmation is also an effective strategy for managing stress, which is especially relevant for mothers juggling multiple responsibilities. Research published in *Psychological Science* found that reflecting on personal beliefs can significantly reduce stress and improve problem-solving skills. For moms dealing with unique challenges, self-affirmation can provide a much-needed mental break, allowing them to manage stress more effectively and build resilience. By adopting this technique they can tackle everyday obstacles with a clearer mindset. Overall, these findings underscore the value of self-affirmation as a practical tool for mothers striving to improve their well-being and navigate the complexities of parenthood.

How to Use Affirmations

1. Identify Key Areas for Growth

Focus on specific aspects of your life where you want to build confidence or shift your mindset. Examples include career aspirations or coping with challenges. Phrases like "I am capable of achieving my goals" can be particularly impactful.

2. Make Them Personal and Positive

Craft affirmations that resonate with you personally and express positive statements. For instance, instead of saying, "I am not afraid," rephrase it as, "I am confident and brave." This encourages a more empowering mindset.

3. Establish a Routine

Incorporate affirmations into your daily routine. Say them in the morning to set a positive tone for the day, repeat them at night to reinforce good feelings, or use them during challenging moments. Consistency is key to solidifying their impact.

4. Replace Negative Thoughts

Use affirmations to counter negative self-talk. If you catch yourself thinking, *I'm not good enough,* consciously replace it with, *I am worthy of success and love.* This cognitive shift can help foster a more positive self-image.

5. Visualize Success

Pair affirmations with visualization techniques. As you recite your affirmations, imagine yourself embodying those qualities or achieving your goals. This can enhance their emotional impact and help manifest your intentions.

6. Stay Patient and Persistent

Remember that change takes time. Be patient with yourself as you practice affirmations and remain persistent. Over time, you may notice positive shifts in your mindset and overall well-being.

Getting Started:

Write down affirmations that resonate with your goals and challenges. Set reminders, like phone alerts or sticky notes, to help you remember to say them throughout the day. By making affirmations a regular part of your life, you can start shifting your mindset and boosting your confidence.

3. MASTERING BREATHWORK

If you've ever been told to take a deep breath in a stressful situation and questioned whether something so simple could truly help, you're not alone. I used to wonder how something as simple as controlled breathing could have such profound effects on emotional balance and nervous system regulation. Here are some answers to common questions that can help clarify how breathwork works and how it might benefit you:

1. What is breathwork?

Breathwork involves various techniques that focus on consciously controlling your breathing patterns. These practices can be used for relaxation, stress management, and personal growth.

2. How does breathwork regulate the nervous system?

Breathwork can impact the autonomic nervous system by transitioning it from the sympathetic (fight or flight) state to the parasympathetic (rest and digest) state. This shift can help reduce stress and promote relaxation.

3. What is stored trauma and how does breathwork help release it?

Stored trauma refers to unresolved emotional experiences or stress that remains in the body. Breathwork can facilitate the release of these stored emotions by promoting deep relaxation and self-awareness, potentially aiding in emotional healing.

4. Are there specific breathwork techniques for emotional balance?

Yes, techniques like diaphragmatic breathing, box breathing, and holotropic breathwork can be particularly effective. Each technique offers different benefits, so exploring various methods can help you find what works best for you.

5. Can breathwork be practiced alone or is guidance necessary?

Breathwork can be practiced independently or with guidance. Beginners might benefit from guided sessions or classes to learn the techniques properly and ensure they are practiced safely.

6. How often should one practice breathwork to see benefits?

The frequency of practice can vary depending on individual needs and goals. Some people find daily practice beneficial while others might practice a few times a week. Consistency is often key to experiencing the full benefits.

7. Are there any risks or contraindications?

While breathwork is generally safe, individuals with certain medical conditions (e.g., respiratory or cardiovascular issues) should consult a healthcare provider before starting. It's also important to practice in a safe environment to avoid hyperventilation or emotional overwhelm.

Understanding these aspects of breathwork can help you approach it with more confidence and clarity.

To incorporate breathwork:

Practice Techniques: Try deep belly breathing, box breathing, or alternate nostril breathing.

Use Daily: Employ these techniques during moments of stress or as part of a calming routine.

Explore Guided Sessions: Use apps or online resources to guide your breathwork practice.

4. VISUALIZATION FOR SUCCESS

Visualization involves creating vivid mental images of goals and desired outcomes. One of the earliest self-help books I encountered was *Think and Grow Rich* by Napoleon Hill (1937), a foundational text in personal development. I was introduced to this book through former mentors in network marketing and it profoundly influenced my approach to success. Without their guidance, I might never have discovered this valuable resource.

Hill (1937) emphasizes the power of visualization, explaining that clearly picturing success aligns the subconscious mind with one's goals. This practice goes beyond mere daydreaming—it is a deliberate mental strategy that prepares and motivates individuals toward success. Regularly visualizing your goals enhances your determination and focus and helps you overcome challenges.

Scientific research also validates the effectiveness of visualization. For example, Cumming and Williams (2013) discovered that imagery is essential for enhancing performance in a variety of fields, such as sports. Their research suggests that visualizing successful outcomes enhances individuals' confidence and performance when they prepare their minds for action. This research emphasizes that visualization is not merely a mental exercise but a practical instrument that transforms abstract aspirations into tangible objectives. Visualization assists individuals in taking tangible actions toward their goals by fostering confidence and establishing a clear mental roadmap.

In essence, visualization serves as more than an imaginative exercise; it is a method of maintaining motivation and direction in the pursuit of long-term goals.

To practice effective visualization:

Establish a Routine: Spend a few minutes each day visualizing your goals.

Engage All Senses: Make the visualization as detailed and sensory-rich as possible.

Focus on Desired Outcomes: Imagine yourself handling a challenging moment with your child with calm and confidence, rather than feeling overwhelmed. Visualize yourself responding with patience and understanding, creating a nurturing environment that supports your child's emotional needs while also allowing you to maintain your own sense of peace.

Action Steps:

Create a Vision Board: Compile images and words that represent your goals and aspirations.

Visualize Regularly: Integrate visualization into your daily routine, ideally in a quiet, distraction-free space.

5. PRIORITIZE QUALITY SLEEP

Quality sleep is vital for learning, memory, and healing, especially after trauma. It helps process new information and supports emotional healing, enhancing your thinking, creativity, and problem-solving skills. In short, good sleep nurtures your brain's ability to heal and adapt, aiding your recovery and overall success.

To enhance sleep quality:

A. Establish a Consistent Schedule
Aim to go to bed and wake up at the same time each day, even on weekends. Consistency reinforces your body's natural circadian rhythm, making it easier to fall asleep and wake up refreshed.

B. Create a Restful Environment
Ensure your sleep environment is conducive to rest by keeping it dark, quiet, and cool. Consider using blackout curtains, earplugs, or white noise machines to minimize disturbances.

C. Use a Weighted Blanket
Incorporate a weighted blanket into your sleep routine. The gentle pressure can help reduce anxiety and promote relaxation, making it easier to fall asleep. Research suggests that weighted blankets can improve sleep quality by providing a calming effect, which may be particularly beneficial for those with anxiety or sensory processing disorders (Davis et al., 2020).

D. Practice Good Sleep Hygiene
Avoid stimulants such as caffeine and nicotine several hours before bedtime. Caffeine, in particular, can disrupt sleep by blocking adenosine, a chemical that promotes sleepiness. Try to limit caffeine intake to the morning hours and opt for herbal teas or decaffeinated beverages in the afternoon and evening.

E. Incorporate Yin Yoga or Other Restorative Practices

Engaging in Yin Yoga or other restorative yoga practices before bed can help calm your mind and body. These gentle stretches and poses promote relaxation and mindfulness, making it easier to transition into sleep (Benson et al., 2014).

F. Dietary Strategies

- Certain foods and supplements can support the natural production of growth hormone, especially when consumed in the evening. Consider the following:
- **Protein-Rich Foods**: Consuming lean protein sources, such as chicken, turkey, fish, and legumes, can provide amino acids that are crucial for growth hormone production. A study by Tam et al. (2020) also highlights that specific amino acid supplements can significantly increase serum hGH levels.
- **Healthy Fats**: Incorporate sources of healthy fats, such as avocados, nuts, and olive oil, to support hormonal balance.

G. Limit Screen Time Before Bed

Exposure to blue light from screens can interfere with melatonin production, making it harder to fall asleep. Aim to turn off electronic devices at least 30–60 minutes before bedtime (Hale & Guan, 2015).

H. Incorporate Physical Activity

Regular physical activity can help regulate sleep patterns and enhance GH production. Aim for at least 30 minutes of moderate exercise on most days, but try to avoid vigorous workouts close to bedtime.

I. Be Mindful of Food and Drink

Avoid heavy meals, alcohol, and excessive fluids before bedtime as these can disrupt sleep. Instead, opt for light snacks if you're hungry.

J. Manage Stress and Anxiety

Incorporate stress-reduction techniques such as mindfulness, meditation, or deep-breathing exercises into your daily routine to help calm your mind before bed.

Action Steps:

1. Design a Bedtime Routine

Incorporate relaxing activities into your pre-sleep routine, such as reading a book, listening to soothing music, or engaging in gentle restorative stretches. This signals to your body that it's time to wind down.

2. Monitor Sleep Patterns

Utilize a sleep tracker or journal to observe your sleep patterns and identify factors that influence your sleep quality. This can help you make informed adjustments to your routine.

3. Engage in Relaxation Techniques

Before bedtime, try engaging in relaxation techniques, such as progressive muscle relaxation or guided imagery. These methods can help ease tension and promote better sleep quality.

4. Limit Naps

If you need to nap during the day, keep it short (20–30 minutes) and avoid napping late in the afternoon. This helps maintain your sleep drive for nighttime rest.

6. CURATING YOUR ENVIRONMENT

Your environment plays a crucial role in shaping your subconscious mind. To create a positive and empowering atmosphere, consider the following strategies:

- **Limit Negative Inputs**: Minimize your exposure to negative news, toxic individuals, and harmful social media. This can help protect your mental space and emotional well-being.
- **Seek Positive Influences**: Surround yourself with uplifting and supportive people who inspire you and encourage personal growth. The energy of those around you can significantly impact your mindset.
- **Engage with Empowering Content**: Choose books, videos, and music that uplift and motivate you. Consuming positive and inspiring content can foster a more optimistic outlook and stimulate personal development.

Action Steps:

1. **Audit Your Environment**: Take a moment to identify sources of negativity in your life. Consider how they affect your mental and emotional state and make a plan to reduce or eliminate them.
2. **Curate Your Media Consumption**: Be intentional about the media you engage with. Opt for content that aligns with your values and supports your growth while opting out of anything that no longer serves you.

(In Chapter 10, we will explore in greater detail how to create a supportive environment that nurtures your well-being.)

7. ENHANCING WITH NEUROPLASTICITY TECHNIQUES

Neuroplasticity—the brain's remarkable ability to adapt and change—can be harnessed to improve cognitive function and overall mental agility. Here are some fun and effective techniques to enhance your brain's plasticity:

- **Engage in Brain Training**: Challenge and stimulate your brain through activities that require critical thinking and problem-solving.

Puzzles, memory games, and strategic games are excellent options. Personally, I love playing chess, solving puzzles, and enjoying a classic game of Scrabble. These activities not only entertain but also promote cognitive flexibility and memory enhancement.

- **Learn a New Skill or Language**: Taking up a new hobby or learning a foreign language can significantly boost neuroplasticity. The process of acquiring new skills forces your brain to create new pathways and connections. Consider trying your hand at painting, playing a musical instrument, or picking up a new language using apps like Duolingo.
- **Connect Socially**: Engaging in meaningful social interactions can stimulate your brain and enhance cognitive resilience. Whether it's joining a club, volunteering, or simply catching up with friends, nurturing relationships can support mental health and cognitive function.
- **Practice Mindfulness and Meditation**: Mindfulness practices and meditation have been shown to increase gray matter in the brain, promoting growth in areas related to memory, emotional regulation, and attention. Incorporate mindfulness exercises or guided meditations into your daily routine to foster a calm and focused mind.

By incorporating these techniques into your routine, you can actively enhance your brain's neuroplasticity and promote long-term cognitive health.

Action Steps:

Adopt New Challenges: Regularly engage in activities that push your cognitive limits.

Practice Mindfulness: Incorporate mindfulness exercises into your daily routine.

Recognizing Progress and Embracing Transformation

As you move through this journey, take a moment to appreciate how far you've come. Every emotional shift is a reminder of your growth. You might notice a new sense of calm in situations that used to overwhelm you—proof of your growing self-awareness.

Positive changes in your behavior are another sign you're on the right path. Maybe you're handling challenges with more patience, building healthier habits, or deepening your relationships. These shifts show the strength you've been cultivating and the progress you're making toward your goals.

Navigating stress more smoothly and facing uncertainty with confidence instead of fear? That's a clear reflection of the hard work you've put in. Each time you overcome a challenge it's proof of your personal growth and the transformation happening in your life.

Celebrate every step forward, no matter how small. These wins highlight your strength and determination, fueling your journey to a more fulfilling life. You're shaping your future with each step, getting closer to the person you're becoming.

Embrace these changes, trust your growth, and remember—you're not just evolving, you're thriving.

CHAPTER 7

Life Happens for You

There are moments in life when everything feels overwhelming. Challenges pile up, one after another, and unresolved past experiences can leave you feeling stuck, almost as if life is happening *to* you rather than *with* you. It's easy to slip into the belief that circumstances are out of your control, trapping you in a cycle of negativity. But what if you could look at things differently? What if, instead of seeing life as a series of obstacles, you saw it as a collection of opportunities to grow and learn?

Take a moment to consider this: You are the author of your own story. It's a powerful shift, realizing that you can rewrite your narrative at any time. This chapter of your life is about that very shift—from feeling like a passive observer, drifting along, to reclaiming your personal power. It starts with reframing how you view challenges. Instead of seeing them as setbacks, what if you saw them as stepping stones to a stronger, more empowered version of you?

Of course, the past can't be erased, nor can the events that have shaped you be ignored. But your current perspective doesn't have to be defined by those events. Think back to a recent challenge, like the COVID-19 pandemic. It's understandable if your first reaction was, "This isn't fair. My life is being upended." Feelings of frustration, fear, and sadness were natural. But what if you took a moment to step back and look at it differently?

You might notice a shift in perspective: "We're all in this together. While this is difficult, I'm still better off than some, and I have the ability to help others." That subtle change in thinking can be transformative. Suddenly, the experience becomes less isolating. You begin to see the world with more gratitude, optimism, and compassion, recognizing the shared humanity in your struggles and those of others.

Reframing isn't just a tool—it's a mindset, a way of turning life's hurdles into opportunities for growth. It invites you to see your challenges in a new light, not as things that hold you back but as experiences that push you forward. As you embrace this shift in thinking you'll begin to break free from the idea that you're powerless in the face of adversity.

Instead, you'll find yourself stepping into your own power, with a renewed sense of purpose and possibility. You'll approach life's difficulties with a greater understanding that you're not just a bystander—you're the hero of your own story. And with that, you have the ability to create a life that's not just about survival but about thriving, growing, and finding fulfillment, even in the face of adversity.

Understanding the Victim Mentality

A victim mentality is rooted in the belief that external factors—other people, circumstances, or fate—are responsible for the difficulties you face. It's characterized by feelings of helplessness, resentment, and a sense of being wronged. While these feelings are valid, staying in this mindset can keep you in this vicious cycle of negativity, focusing on what you can't control rather than what you can.

Signs of a victim mentality might include:

1. Blaming Others: Constantly pointing fingers and attributing your struggles to others or external circumstances, rather than reflecting on your own role or actions.

2. Self-Pity: Regularly feeling that life is unfair and dwelling on how you're being wronged, instead of focusing on solutions or taking charge of your situation.

3. Hopelessness: Believing that nothing will ever improve and feeling trapped in a cycle of negativity and despair, as if you're stuck in a never-ending struggle.

4. Feeling Powerless: A deep-seated sense that you can't change anything in your life, leading to passivity and a belief that you're at the mercy of fate or others.

5. Negative Self-Talk: Engaging in harsh, critical self-talk that keeps you feeling inadequate and reinforces a sense of helplessness, eroding your self-confidence.

6. Avoiding Responsibility: Shifting blame for your problems or mistakes onto others, instead of owning up to your actions and learning from them. This can lead to a lack of personal growth and unresolved issues.

7. Overgeneralizing: Taking one bad experience and letting it color your entire outlook, believing that because something went wrong once, everything else is bound to fail as well.

The Power of Reframing: Trial to Triumph

Reframing is like putting on new glasses to view life's challenges from a more positive and empowering perspective. It's not about denying the reality of difficulties but about changing how you interpret and respond to them. By reframing, you can shift from feeling powerless to embracing your own strength and choices.

One experience that perfectly illustrates the power of reframing is when I used to feel devastated after dropping my kids off at school. Even the smallest mishap—like forgetting a lunch bag—could trigger a torrent of frustration and despair. I'd drive away, my heart heavy, caught in a storm of nagging and shouting, all while unresolved trauma raged within me. As soon as I was alone, the tears would come, streaming down my face in a flood of anguish. I was haunted by fears that I was failing as a mother, that my outbursts were leaving scars on my children. The weight of this guilt felt unbearable and I worried that my moments of turmoil might be doing irreparable harm to their lives.

These moments were painful and made me question my worth. However, through the practice of reframing, I learned to approach these challenges differently. Instead of viewing these situations as evidence of my failure, I began to see them as opportunities for growth. With techniques like mindfulness and self-reflection, I practiced pausing in moments of frustration and shifting my focus from guilt to understanding. I learned to ask myself, "What can I learn from this moment?" or "How can I handle this situation better next time?"

This change in perspective allowed me to transform guilt and regret into lessons in self-compassion and resilience. I began to forgive myself for not being a perfect mom and saw each challenge as a way to grow both personally and as a mother. Reframing not only aided my healing but also helped me create a more positive and nurturing environment for my family. I began responding to my children with more patience, showing them how to handle their own struggles with grace and strength, which, in turn, improved their emotional responses.

As I practiced reframing, I noticed a shift in my behavior as well. I was able to manage stress and face obstacles with greater ease. For example, when I encountered uncertainty, I approached it with curiosity and confidence rather than fear, knowing that every challenge was an opportunity to build my resilience. Each time I navigated a difficult situation with a positive mindset I felt a sense of validation. It became clear that my efforts were creating meaningful change.

Reframing has since become an essential tool in my life, not just for handling day-to-day struggles but for cultivating long-term emotional resilience. Each small victory serves as a reminder of my strength and capacity for growth. Celebrate every step forward, no matter how small, because these shifts mark a path toward a more empowered and fulfilling life. Reframing doesn't just change how you see the world—it changes how you engage with it, allowing you to thrive, not just survive.

How Reframing Can Transform Your Feelings and Thoughts

Integrating the Internal Family Systems (IFS) model with Neuro-Linguistic Programming (NLP) makes the process of reframing even more powerful. It's not just about changing the narrative; it's about transforming how different parts of yourself—exiles, managers, and firefighters—perceive and respond to experiences.

Exiles: These parts hold deep emotional pain, shame, or fear from past traumas. Reframing through IFS invites exiles to view experiences through a more compassionate lens. Instead of seeing your struggles as failures, this approach helps exiles recognize them as courageous steps toward healing. By contextualizing these experiences you offer them understanding and support, which can ease their emotional burden.

Managers: These parts strive to control your environment and behavior to avoid pain. Reframing helps managers adopt a more compassionate perspective, seeing struggles as integral parts of your growth journey rather than personal shortcomings. This shift allows them to relax their tight grip on control and embrace a gentler approach, fostering internal harmony.

Firefighters: These parts react impulsively to distract from or numb the pain of exiles, often through avoidance or emotional outbursts. Reframing offers firefighters a new way to manage distress. By helping them approach challenges with a more balanced perspective, they can find calm and resolve without relying on immediate distractions or reactions.

Reframing does more than just change your thoughts; it deeply impacts how you feel about your experiences. It's about shifting your perspective so that situations feel less burdensome and more manageable. This shift helps lighten the emotional load and creates a more supportive and harmonious internal environment.

In Internal Family Systems (IFS) therapy, we recognize different aspects of your psyche as parts—like exiles (which carry painful memories), managers (which try to control and prevent discomfort), and firefighters (which soothe immediate distress). Reframing the perspectives these parts hold can help ease their burdens and create a more balanced internal state.

When you integrate Neuro-Linguistic Programming (NLP) into your personal development journey, the transformation becomes even more impactful. NLP helps you understand and reshape the thought and behavior patterns that drive your experiences. Techniques like anchoring, reframing, and visualization are designed to shift emotional responses and break habitual thought patterns, making it easier to manage your emotions and create meaningful change.

By combining Internal Family Systems (IFS) with NLP, you gain a robust toolkit for personal growth. IFS offers insights into understanding and harmonizing your internal parts while NLP equips you with practical methods for reshaping thoughts and emotions. Together, they foster deeper self-awareness and emotional resilience, paving the way for a more balanced, fulfilling inner life.

This approach offers not just clarity but also the confidence to take control of your emotional and mental landscape.

Steps to Embrace Personal Power and Agency

1. Acknowledge Your Feelings:

Recognize and accept your emotions without judgment. It's okay to feel hurt, angry, or sad. These are natural responses to life's challenges. The goal is not to dwell in these feelings but to use them as a springboard for change.

2. Identify Limiting Beliefs:

Explore the beliefs underpinning your victim mentality. Do you believe you're incapable, that life is unfair, or that you have no control? These beliefs, often formed in childhood, can be deeply ingrained but are not set in stone. Question them. Are they absolutely true? What evidence do you have to the contrary?

3. Reframe Your Narrative:

Start telling yourself a different story. Instead of, "This always happens to me," try, "What can I learn from this situation?" or "How can I turn this around?" Reframing shifts your focus from what's wrong to what's possible.

4. Take Responsibility:

Own your choices and actions as a key step in reclaiming your power. This doesn't mean blaming yourself for everything but recognizing your role in responding to life's challenges. Taking responsibility helps you regain control.

5. Set Intentions and Take Action:

Shift from passive to active by setting clear intentions and breaking down goals into manageable steps. Start taking action, no matter how small. Each step forward is a testament to your personal power.

6. Cultivate Resilience:

Life will continue to throw challenges your way, but your response is within your control. Cultivate resilience by practicing self-compassion, maintaining a growth mindset, and surrounding yourself with supportive people. Resilience is about bouncing back and moving forward, even when things get tough.

Overcoming Resistance: Navigating the Challenges

Shifting from a victim mentality to embracing personal power is a courageous journey, yet it's not without its challenges. If this mindset has been a long-standing part of your life, you might encounter internal resistance in the form of doubt, fear, or guilt. Acknowledging these feelings is the first step toward overcoming them. It's crucial to approach this process with persistence and self-compassion.

Doubt: Trusting Your Ability to Change

Doubt often creeps in when we consider making significant changes. It's completely natural to question your ability to control your life and create the future you desire. However, remember that change is a process filled with ups and downs. Every individual who has successfully transformed their lives has encountered moments of uncertainty. The key is to view doubt not as a sign of failure but as a natural part of stepping outside your comfort zone. Embrace it as a signal that you are pushing against your boundaries and growing in the process.

Self-compassion can significantly mitigate feelings of doubt. By being kind to yourself and recognizing that everyone struggles with self-doubt, you can cultivate a more positive and forgiving mindset. Remind yourself that every small step you take is a testament to your courage and determination.

Fear: Taking Small Steps Forward

Fear of the unknown can paralyze you, causing you to hesitate when action is most critical. To combat this, break your journey down into small, manageable steps. Avoid getting caught up in the big picture and focus on today. Each small victory builds confidence and momentum, making the path ahead feel less daunting.

Celebrate each step as progress, no matter how minor it may seem. This practice of acknowledging your achievements reinforces your sense of agency and strengthens your belief in your abilities. Celebrating small wins can improve motivation and foster a sense of accomplishment, helping you move past fear.

Guilt: Choosing a Healthier Path

Leaving behind a victim mentality can evoke feelings of guilt, particularly if you've grown accustomed to receiving sympathy or support in that role. It's important to recognize that choosing to empower yourself is not an act of abandonment; rather, it's a decision to pursue a healthier and more fulfilling path for yourself and those around you.

Accept that personal power benefits you and your relationships. By controlling your life, you create the capacity to support others more effectively. Self-empowerment can lead to improved interpersonal relationships as empowered individuals tend to communicate more openly and assertively.

The Journey to Empowerment

Shifting from a victim attitude to embracing personal power is a gradual process that includes ups and downs. As I share my story, I want to acknowledge that I don't have a complete resolution and that's perfectly fine. I still have my challenges and uncertainties, but I've realized that I'm learning to negotiate the intricacies of my life with strength and perseverance. Maybe I'm just two steps ahead of someone else, but those steps are important and I welcome the lessons they teach.

This road requires patience, perseverance, and a steadfast dedication to self-development. Despite the weight of my past, I recognize my potential for substantial change. Each step I take reclaims more of my authority, reminding me that I am in control of my life. It's crucial also to remember that growth isn't always linear; it may be chaotic and unpredictable. Some days, I stand tall and confident, and others, I doubt my decisions. Nonetheless, I refuse to allow self-doubt to determine my destiny. Instead, I choose to accept the pain, knowing it will help me develop.

The fear of change is real, but there comes a point when the pain of staying where you are hurts even more. Growth might be tough, but staying stuck only deepens the ache. - Farrah Domaoan

Remember, what happened to you isn't your fault, but how you respond to it is your responsibility. It is your reaction to your circumstances that defines you, not your background. Realize that you have the ability to rewrite your story with conviction and be confident in that capability.

By embracing your own power and learning to reframe your experiences, you not only alter your life but serve as an example to others. Your story may teach them that they, too, can overcome obstacles and forge their own road to success. It's a poignant reminder that we're all works in progress and that's where our strength rests.

"Used Sanitary Pads"

I recall the muffled laughter that trailed behind me, the sidelong stares, and the whispers that echoed through the apartment complex. "Mabaho," they sneered, the Tagalog word for stinky. At first I tried to ignore their taunts, convincing myself that their words had no power over me. But as the ridicule intensified, I began to internalize their remarks, accepting the belief that I was fundamentally flawed.

My neglect of self-care was deeply rooted in trauma, a tangled accumulation of anguish and humiliation that stretched back to my earliest memories. This pain lurked in the shadows of my mind, buried beneath layers of denial and suppression.

In the aftermath of that harrowing sexual violation, I retreated into myself, constructing walls around my heart to fend off further pain. The simple act of bathing became a source of dread; the sensation of water on my skin triggered visceral reactions of fear and aversion. My school uniforms were stained and reeking of sweat, which lay neglected at the bottom of my dresser drawers, a stark reflection of my inability to meet even the most basic of needs.

Imagine a closet—a place that's supposed to hold our everyday things. But for me, it held secrets. I was hiding old, used sanitary pads in the back of my dresser, burying them beneath layers of clothes. I couldn't throw them out because discarding them would mean facing something I wasn't ready to confront. This wasn't about the physical items; it was about my story—the shame, the trauma, the parts of me I believed were too messy, too ugly to look at. Their existence wasn't just about neglect; it embodied the paralyzing fear that held me captive. So they remained hidden in the dark, their faint odor a small price to pay for avoiding any potential confrontation with the source of my torment.

I was hiding painful parts of myself, trying to discard them in the same way. But these parts just didn't go away. They lingered, lurking, influencing every role I chose to play in my life.

The burden of neglecting self-care loomed over my childhood, shaping the very core of who I was becoming. It was more than just physical illness or an exhausted appearance; it penetrated deep into my being, sowing seeds of doubt, self-pity, and self-loathing that flourished with alarming tenacity.

At nine years old, I grappled with feelings of unworthiness that stifled any flicker of hope within me. I watched as my peers navigated self-care practices effortlessly and I couldn't help but wonder why I was incapable of the same. The whispers of self-doubt grew louder each day, infecting my mind and heart.

Every morning felt like a battlefield as I confronted not only the physical pain of neglect but also the mental weight of feeling inadequate and unlovable. It was as if I bore the weight of the world. And when I looked in the mirror, the reflection was a harsh reminder of how neglecting self-care had scarred my young psyche.

However, as I got older, something unexpected happened. The allure of the influencer world captivated me as I desperately tried to regain some control over my life. I became paradoxically obsessed with self-care; I was still trying to hide, but now I was hiding in the other way. I lost myself in painstakingly planned routines—skincare practices that made it difficult to distinguish between ritualistic avoidance and self-love. I purchased a slew of items, each with a glimmering promise of well-being, all with the intention of concealing my emotional troubles under layers of beauty.

I created an idealized persona in the radiance of social media because I thought that if I could just put on a positive front, I could get rid of the suffering that plagued me. However, the same concerns still lurked under the surface, saying that no amount of polish could remove the wounds I bore. The glitz of it all was euphoric, but the process of making myself seem good turned into a prison in and of itself.

It felt almost dissociative as I became lost in my need for approval and grappled with the duality of my identity. The struggle to embody the perfect influencer masked the turmoil within me, leaving me teetering between hiding and healing. Despite the deep sadness that lingered beneath my well-manicured exterior, I found solace in a society that seemed to value beauty above all else.

But beneath the surface, the old fears lingered, whispering that no amount of self-care could truly shield me from the pain I had endured. In striving to cultivate a polished exterior I often lost sight of the deeper healing I desperately needed. The weight of my past remained; a shadow I couldn't fully escape, even as I plastered on smiles and shared my newfound skincare routine with the world.

CHAPTER 8

Self-Care Unplugged: Am I Being True to Myself?

In today's wellness-saturated world, we're constantly bombarded with messages like: *"To be a better mom, a happier person, and a more fulfilled individual, you must prioritize self-care. In fact, putting self-care first is putting your children first."* While well-intentioned, this perspective barely scratches the surface of what it means to truly show up as a better mother, a happier individual, and a fulfilled human being.

The Superficiality and Limitations of Mainstream Self-Care

The current narrative often reduces self-care to surface-level activities such as bubble baths, spa days, binge-watching Netflix, and 'me-time. 'While I have indulged in these practices myself, often relying on them for the wrong reasons, they can provide only momentary relief or enjoyment. This approach implies that simple indulgences can transform one's well-being, yet they fail to address the deeper, more complex needs essential for lasting fulfillment and genuine personal growth. As discussed in Chapter 3, unresolved trauma is persistent emotional pain and stress that superficial self-care methods cannot undo. True self-care demands deep, sometimes uncomfortable, inner work, requiring an understanding of the impact of trauma on mental health, meaningful self-reflection, and a commitment to genuine healing rather than relying on quick fixes.

Real Transformation Requires More Than Pampering

I used to think that a quick hour of "me time"—mindlessly strolling the aisles of Target or getting a manicure—would be enough to make me a better mom. Don't get me wrong; those moments of self-care are important, but being truly present and resilient for your children—and for yourself—requires more than just a temporary recharge. Being emotionally available and authentically engaged every day is where the money is at. Real growth and connection come from consistent effort, not just a fleeting moment of self-care. It comes from actively engaging in your own healing and growth journey, which may involve confronting past traumas, setting healthy boundaries, nurturing your emotional well-being, or challenging deep-seated beliefs. Real self-care is about embracing who you truly are, flaws and all.

- **Resilience and Presence**: True self-care involves building emotional resilience by addressing the psychological impact of triggers and stressors. In Chapter 4, we explore how common triggers affect moms and the importance of understanding and managing them to foster emotional stability.
- **Deeper Work**: Engaging in self-care means addressing past traumas, setting and maintaining healthy boundaries, and working on personal development. This includes creating a personalized stress plan (Chapter 9) that identifies what these stressors are and developing strategies to manage them.

Reimagining Self-Care

Let's rethink self-care. It's not merely an itinerary of spa days or weekend retreats; it's a transformative journey of self-discovery and acceptance. It's about becoming the best version of you, rather than conforming to societal expectations of what it means to be a "better" mom. These pressures might include unrealistic standards of perfection, constant comparisons to others, or the need to meet every external expectation. True self-care is deeply personal and profoundly redemptive, touching on a soul-level connection with you. As the quote goes, "What you're seeking is seeking you." This means that when you align your self-care practices with your innermost desires, you naturally attract the joy, fulfillment, contentment and longevity you seek. However, past traumas and the demands of motherhood can sometimes cause us to lose sight of our true north.

So, what is it that you truly desire or want at your core? By tuning into what genuinely nourishes your spirit and aligns with your deepest values—what we might call soul-level alignment—you create a powerful resonance that attracts those very things into your life. This alignment is about connecting with your core values and deepest desires and it's grounded in practical, actionable steps rather than any mystical or esoteric ideas. It fosters a deep, lasting transformation that enriches your existence. Your authentic self-care practices act as a guiding light, leading you toward a more meaningful and fulfilled life. Remember, what drew you to this book is its practical approach to self-care and these principles are designed to be both actionable and transformative.

While bubble baths and other specific physical self-care activities are rightfully comforting, it's important to focus on the deeper, more meaningful aspects of self-care. By viewing it as an ongoing process of growth and acceptance, we recognize that it's more than just tasks—it's a path to personal development, self-discovery and emotional resilience. This approach helps us move beyond external pressures, fostering a deeper understanding of ourselves and aligning with what truly resonates with our values. Committing to this authentic pursuit of self-care supports profound growth, greater joy, and a healthier, more enduring life.

Nurturing Self-Worth: Escaping the Validation Trap

Have you ever posted a picture on Instagram, eagerly checking your phone for likes and comments? Perhaps it was a family photo or a moment when you treated yourself to a day out. But as the minutes passed, the number of likes fell short of your expectations, diminishing that small moment of joy.

If you can relate, you're not alone. The craving for external validation often serves as a coping mechanism for deeper feelings of inadequacy or self-doubt. Social media, with its likes, comments, and endless comparisons, becomes a fleeting source of approval.

It's crucial to understand that the success or happiness of others does not detract from our own potential for joy and fulfillment. Tying our self-worth to likes and others' achievements fosters a zero-sum mindset, positioning us as competitors instead of collaborators. Instead, we can celebrate others' achievements as sources of inspiration. By breaking free from this mentality we allow ourselves to flourish without feeling threatened by those around us.

But what is it about those likes and comments that draws us in so powerfully? Why do we often feel just as empty afterward, if not more, despite the temporary high they provide?

The Brain's Response to Social Media Validation

When you receive a like or a positive comment on your post, your brain releases dopamine, a neurotransmitter associated with pleasure and reward.

It's similar to the delight of biting into your favorite dessert; for a brief moment, everything feels a little brighter. This dopamine hit signals your brain, "This feels good—do it again."

However, just like with any quick fix, the satisfaction from these likes is like a vapor. Your brain begins to crave more, leading to an increasing dependence on external validation. As a result, your sense of self-worth becomes tied to how the outside world responds to you.

Why External Validation Feels Comforting—But Ultimately Incomplete

Think back to a time when you felt particularly vulnerable—perhaps after a long, exhausting day where nothing seemed to go right. You posted something on social media, hoping the notifications would provide a boost. Each like offered a moment of relief, a sense of being seen or appreciated, but when the notifications slowed down, that good feeling evaporated, leaving you with the same doubts and worries.

For mothers with unresolved trauma, this craving for external validation can run even deeper. Traumatic experiences, especially from childhood or early adulthood, profoundly shape your self-perception. If you've never fully healed from those wounds, you might rely on others to affirm that you're good enough, loved, or worthy. In this context, social media can act as a substitute for genuine affirmation, even if only temporarily.

The truth is, depending on external validation—whether from Instagram or people in your daily life—creates an emotional imbalance. The more you seek approval from outside the more disconnected you become from the only validation that truly lasts: the validation that comes from within.

Transition: From External Approval to Self-Awareness

So how do you break this cycle? **The first step is self-awareness.** Recognizing when and why you're seeking external validation can be the key to unlocking deeper emotional healing and well-being. It's about shifting your focus from what others think of you to how you feel about yourself. This is where the practice of self-care transforms from surface-level indulgence into something far more profound: nurturing your internal self-worth.

Self-Awareness: The Foundation of Lasting Self-Care

Becoming self-aware means recognizing the patterns that lead you to seek validation from others. It involves understanding the triggers—like moments of self-doubt, stress, or comparison—that push you to post a picture or check for likes. It's about pausing long enough to ask yourself, **"What am I really seeking here?"**

Self-awareness empowers you to step back from the dopamine-fueled chase of approval and look inward. When you cultivate this awareness, you start recognizing that those moments of scrolling, posting, and waiting for feedback are often tied to unmet emotional needs. Maybe you're seeking connection because you're feeling isolated or maybe you want affirmation because you're feeling unsure about your role as a mother.

Practical Steps for Developing Self-Awareness

1. Notice Your Triggers:

The next time you feel the urge to check your phone for likes or post something on social media, pause and ask yourself: **"Why am I doing this? What am I hoping to feel?"** This simple act of questioning can bring powerful awareness to habits that may otherwise feel automatic.

For example, if you're posting a picture of your child's achievement, ask yourself if you're sharing out of joy or because you're hoping others will affirm your parenting.

2. Practice Mindful Posting:

Before you post, take a moment to check in with your emotions. Are you feeling happy, anxious, lonely, or proud? Acknowledging your feelings can help you approach social media more mindfully, turning it into a tool for authentic expression rather than a source of validation.

3. Set Boundaries for Social Media:

Consider setting limits on how much time you spend online. Designate specific times for social media use and consciously disconnect afterward. By creating intentional boundaries you give yourself space to focus on the present, nurturing real-life connections and self-care practices.

4. Journal for Internal Validation:

Keep a journal where you write down things you're proud of—without needing anyone else's validation. Whether it's small accomplishments from your day or reflections on how you handled a tough situation, this practice strengthens your internal validation muscle. Over time, your brain will begin to seek affirmation from within, not from the outside world.

From Self-Care to Self-Awareness: A New Path to Valuing Yourself

What if we viewed self-care not just as a checklist of activities but as a state of being? True self-care emerges from embracing self-awareness—understanding your unique needs, recognizing your triggers, and honoring your boundaries. It's not about fixing something broken because you are not broken. Often, we yearn for getaways, believing a change of scenery will alleviate our overwhelm. But are we truly seeking rest or are we attempting to escape unresolved parts of us?

When we perceive self-care solely as an external remedy—a retreat or a spa day—we may fall into the misconception that we need to improve ourselves. However, self-care isn't about fleeing from our lives or ourselves; it's about cultivating the inner awareness and peace that allow us to show up fully, even in the hardest moments. We don't need to run from our challenges or numb our emotions. Instead, true self-care means leaning into self-compassion, trusting ourselves to navigate life's difficulties, and recognizing that we are enough, exactly as we are.

As you begin to build self-awareness you'll find that the need for external validation diminishes. You'll learn to celebrate your own worth, independent of likes and comments. This shift—though gradual—empowers you to practice self-care from a place of abundance rather than lack. It's not about indulgence or quick fixes; it's about honoring your needs on deeper emotional and physical levels. By breaking free from the validation trap, you reclaim your emotional health and lay a more stable foundation for lasting well-being—one that transcends into new heights of longevity.

The real work lies not in escape but in the daily choices we make to align with our values, honor our needs, and stay connected to our authentic selves. The more aware you become of your patterns the more empowered you are to change them. And that, in itself, is a profound form of radical self-care—loving yourself in every moment, not just the easy ones.

EMOTIONAL CHECK-IN

You're more than halfway through this book—how are you feeling about everything so far? As you reflect on the insights and practices we've explored together, consider what beliefs are shaping your perspective. What do you hold to be true about yourself, your worth, and your experiences? If you're unsure, that's perfectly okay. Exploring these beliefs is an essential part of your journey.

The Deeper Work of Healing

Self-awareness is truly the heart and cornerstone of effective self-care. It connects you to your beliefs and helps you understand how unresolved trauma can influence your reactions in daily life. Think about it: are your beliefs rooted in love and acceptance or are they clouded by doubt and criticism? Taking the time to examine this can reveal so much about your emotional landscape.

Now let's take it a step further. **What about the stories you've told yourself for so long?** It's time to throw those out the window. The person you thought you were in the past—she's still there, in the background, cheering you on as you say goodbye to those outdated narratives. Thank her for the lessons she brought you, but recognize that you're ready to move forward, creating a new story rooted in self-acceptance and growth.

What old beliefs no longer serve you? How does it feel to imagine saying goodbye to them? Remember: **You are more than your past. You are capable of growth and change.**

In this age of social media, where the number of likes and comments can easily sway our sense of self-worth, nurturing this awareness becomes even more crucial. It gives you the strength to navigate challenges with grace and make choices that truly prioritize your well-being.

As we dive deeper into the practice of self-care we'll explore approaches that go beyond quick fixes. Healing is perhaps the most profound form of self-care as it involves compassionately addressing the roots of stress, guilt, feelings of unworthiness, shame, and humiliation. This journey requires courage and recognizing these emotions is a beautiful first step toward a renewed self. By gently confronting past wounds and allowing yourself to be vulnerable, you can reclaim ownership of your healing journey.

As Brené Brown wisely reminds us, **"Vulnerability is the birthplace of innovation, creativity, and change."** Embracing your vulnerability not only fosters personal growth but also empowers you to reframe your experiences, reinforcing that you are capable of meaningful change. You'll find that your past doesn't have to define you; instead, it becomes a part of your story that enriches your journey.

By cultivating self-awareness and embracing vulnerability you open yourself to deeper connections with yourself and those around you. This shift transforms your approach to self-care into one that genuinely honors who you are at your core.

To begin this transformation, consider writing a letter to your past self. Express gratitude for the lessons learned and gently let go of the beliefs that no longer serve you.

I want you to imagine this: It's early in the morning. The house is still quiet and you're sitting at the kitchen table with a warm cup of tea in your hands. The light is soft and, for the first time in a while, there's space to just *be*. In that moment, you take a breath. Maybe you haven't really stopped to breathe like this in days, maybe longer. And as you sit there, something shifts. The weight you've been carrying—the worries, the old hurts, the pressure to be everything to everyone—starts to feel a little lighter. There's room to reflect, to reimagine the story you've been telling yourself.

Later, when your child runs up to you—frustrated or excited—you notice that something's changed. Instead of reacting out of exhaustion or stress, you're able to be present. You really hear them. You listen intently, and in that moment, you realize you're no longer carrying the same old weight. The unresolved sorrow, the need to meet every demand—they don't control how you show up anymore. You've started to shift, to let go of the past in ways that make you more authentic, more grounded in who you truly are. And that's what your children feel when they're with you now—your calm, your resilience, your ability to be fully there with them.

This is the journey of **Reimagined Motherhood: Untriggered**. It's not about having all the answers or never getting frustrated; it's about recognizing those moments when you used to fall into old patterns—whether it was a spilled glass of milk or a tantrum—and responding with more ease. Instead of reacting, you take a breath, pause, and choose a different way forward. You're no longer driven by frustration or the need to control. You're learning to navigate these moments with more awareness, with patience, with love and grace.

And as you continue on this path, the changes become more visible. The relationship with your children starts to shift too. There's more connection, more space for real conversation. You find that emotions can flow more freely without the tension that used to sit just beneath the surface. Your children start to see you as someone who's patient and steady, even in the chaos of daily life. And in that, they're learning from you—how to be resilient, how to handle life's challenges, how to self-validate and how to accept themselves just as they are.

Every time you choose to care for yourself in this way—by pausing, by breathing, by reflecting—you're breaking old generational patterns and creating deeper, more meaningful connections. This is the essence of **Untriggered**: not just managing the day-to-day but truly being present for yourself and your children, building relationships that are grounded in self-acceptance, in your truth, which no longer is bounded by the past.

CHAPTER 9

Calm Blueprint

Not preparing in advance is essentially setting yourself up for failure. Stress is an inevitable part of life and while it can be challenging, it isn't always negative. But what if you had a plan in place to manage stress before it managed you? That's where your Stress Plan comes in! Think of your Stress Plan as your emotional first aid kit, filled with tools and strategies you can reach for whenever you feel stress levels rising.

As Stephen Covey wisely stated, "Begin with the end in mind" (Covey, 1989). This principle encourages individuals to envision their desired outcomes, which is precisely what your Stress Plan allows you to do. Imagine it as a customizable resource, designed to fit your life perfectly—a collection of proven techniques that help you maintain composure and equilibrium, regardless of the challenges life throws at you. From journaling to a quick breathing exercise, your plan will serve as your go-to resource for finding balance in stressful situations.

Once you've created your Stress Plan, keep it visible—on your fridge, in your planner, or as a note on your phone. Those yellow sticky notes are the best. Place them everywhere! Use it whenever you feel stress creeping in. Remember, having a plan is a proactive step toward managing stress and maintaining emotional balance. It's important to recognize that not all stress is detrimental; eustress, or positive stress, can motivate you to take on challenges and push yourself toward personal growth (Selye, 1976).

Regularly review and update your plan as needed; be kind and give yourself grace. Stress is a normal part of life and your Stress Plan is there to help you handle it along the way. Embracing both eustress and distress within your plan can empower you to navigate life's ups and downs with a more balanced perspective.

Creating your Stress Plan isn't about achieving a stress-free life; it's about equipping yourself with effective tools and strategies. Embrace it as a journey of self-discovery and celebrate each step you take toward managing stress. You've got this!

Interactive Exercise: Guided Journaling Prompt - Your Stress Plan

Identifying Your Stressors

1. What are the top three things that consistently stress you out?
Reflect on your daily or weekly routine and jot down the common stressors.

2. How do you usually feel when you're stressed?
Describe the physical and emotional signs that let you know you're stressed.

3. When do you experience the most stress during the day or week?
Note any specific times or situations that trigger your stress.

4. What recent events or situations have caused you the most stress?
Identify recent examples to understand your stress patterns better.

Figuring Out What Calms You Down

5. What activities or practices have helped you relax in the past?
List any techniques or activities that have previously helped you de-stress.

6. Who or what brings you comfort during stressful times?
Think about people, pets, or things that make you feel better when you're stressed.

7. How does your body respond to stress relief techniques?
Reflect on any physical changes or feelings you notice when you use stress-relief strategies.

8. What small, simple things can you do to take care of yourself when you're feeling overwhelmed?
Consider quick, accessible activities that can offer immediate relief.

Creating a Go-To List of Stress-Busting Activities

9. What are your top five favorite stress-relief activities?
List activities that you genuinely enjoy and that help you relax.

10. How can you incorporate these activities into your daily or weekly routine?
Plan how you can regularly engage in these activities to maintain balance.

11. What self-care practices can you add to your routine that might help you manage stress better?
Explore new self-care ideas or habits to include in your lifestyle.

12. What can you do to create a calming environment at home?
Think about changes you can make to your living space that can contribute to a more peaceful atmosphere.

Final Touches

13. How will you remind yourself to use your stress plan when you're feeling overwhelmed?

Develop a strategy for keeping your stress plan visible and accessible.

14. What steps can you take to ensure you stick to your stress plan even during busy times?

Consider ways to maintain your stress plan's effectiveness during hectic periods.

15. How will you evaluate the effectiveness of your stress plan?

Decide how you will assess whether your plan is working and make adjustments as needed.

CHAPTER 10

Creating a Supportive Environment

Close your eyes for a moment and picture yourself in a room filled with people who truly understand you—who empathize with your struggles, celebrate your successes, and are there to offer a helping hand whenever you need it. That's the transformative power of a supportive environment. Such a community is not just comforting; it embodies the principles of trauma-informed care, which focus on understanding the impact of trauma and creating spaces that foster healing and resilience. In these supportive settings, individuals feel safe and valued, cultivating trust and encouraging personal growth and recovery (Treatment, C. F. S. A., 2014).

For mothers on their healing journey, trauma-informed care is particularly significant. According to the Substance Abuse and Mental Health Services Administration (SAMHSA), the six key principles of a trauma-informed approach are:

1. **Safety**: Ensuring a physically and emotionally safe environment.

2. **Trustworthiness and Transparency**: Building trust through clear communication and expectations.

3. **Peer Support**: Encouraging connections with others who share similar experiences.

4. **Collaboration and Mutuality**: Involving mothers in their healing processes and decision-making.

5. **Empowerment, Voice, and Choice**: Promoting autonomy and ensuring that mothers feel heard and respected.

6. **Cultural and Historical Awareness**: Recognizing and addressing the unique cultural and historical contexts of individuals.

These principles empower mothers to acknowledge their experiences while providing them with the tools to break the cycle of trauma. By prioritizing emotional well-being, trauma-informed care enables mothers to cultivate healthier relationships with their children and create a more resilient family dynamic.

If you're a plant mom, you might really connect with this analogy. Think of your support network as a lively collection of houseplants. Each person in your life—family, friends, mentors—adds their own unique touch, much like different types of plants. Some are like sturdy monsteras, giving you a solid foundation and reliable support, while others are like cheerful rubber plants, bringing color and joy to your days.

When you find someone who's been by your side through life's circus—a sister, a mom, or a best friend—hold on to her. She's like a resilient snake plant, offering steady support no matter what. Look for friends who can walk alongside you through shared experiences, like navigating the challenges of "mom life" together. These friendships are like nurturing pothos vines, helping you grow and flourish through all the seasons of life.

As you've seen throughout this book, I've relied on different tools to guide me along the way. One surprising yet powerful tool is something as simple as tuning into the right podcast—one that truly resonates with you. It's like listening to a trusted friend who offers just the right words of comfort and clarity when you need them most. One of my favorites is *Let It Be Easy* with Susie Moore, which perfectly captures this feeling. The show highlights the importance of embracing simplicity and ease in both relationships and daily life. It beautifully aligns with the idea of surrounding yourself with people who make life feel effortless—where you can be completely yourself, free of judgment. Their presence, like a blooming peace lily, brings brightness, joy, and lightness to your days.

When you find a friend who can share both laughter and tears with you in the same conversation, treasure them deeply. This kind of friend is a rare gem, someone who truly understands and supports you through all of life's emotional highs and lows. She enriches your life, offering both comfort and joy, much like a nurturing fern that adds warmth and depth to your life's garden. She becomes a vital part of your support network, helping you navigate the journey with empathy and love.

Creating a nurturing environment within you begins with self-compassion. Let go of self-judgment and embrace your feelings with kindness. Replace self-criticism with understanding and validation. Encourage open, honest conversations with yourself and let go of fear. Just as a cherished plant corner makes your home feel cozy and alive, a supportive and loving environment helps you grow and thrive. Celebrate the wonderful connections you make, knowing they reflect your strength and resilience.

Navigating Medication and Mental Health: A Personal Reflection

The Limitations of Traditional Treatments

Dealing with mental health issues can sometimes seem like a complex path involving medication and conventional therapies. Medication can sometimes give a quick solution, but it usually only offers short-term relief and fails to address the underlying problems.

I recall going to the doctor multiple times, each visit bringing up different symptoms and worries. However, it felt like every appointment concluded with the same prescription and a recommendation to go back on medication. The doctor's approach, which solely focused on a "differential diagnosis" of anxiety, led to a continuous cycle of medication that failed to address my evolving symptoms. This method frequently came across as dismissive, leaving me in search of a more thorough understanding.

A really intense moment happened during a visit with my spouse when the doctor brought up the idea of referring us to a psychiatrist. I sat there squeezing his hand as I struggled to hold back tears, sensing that the advice provided no real alternatives and made me feel insignificant and overlooked. This moment reminded me of my childhood, when I often felt ignored and overlooked, heightening my feelings of frustration and helplessness. However, this experience revealed a hidden blessing. It served as a wake-up call, highlighting gaps in my care and inspiring me to take a more proactive role in my mental health journey.

Traditional Western medicine is excellent with its scientific methods and has made huge strides, but it sometimes has trouble addressing the more intangible aspects of mental health. Although these scientific approaches hold significant importance, they primarily concentrate on observable and measurable aspects, potentially overlooking broader social, cultural, and emotional factors.

The Complexities of Modern Addictions

People often view addiction narrowly, primarily focusing on substances like alcohol and drugs. However, it can also manifest in various behaviors, such as compulsive shopping, overeating, and excessive social media use. The latter can create a constant need for validation and comparison, significantly impacting mental health and productivity. Compulsive shopping, or oniomania, is a prime example of this modern addiction. It reflects an uncontrollable urge to shop, often driven by emotional distress, and can act as a way to cope rather than addressing deeper issues.

During the pandemic, I found myself in a similar situation. As stores closed and then gradually reopened, I went on a shopping spree, buying thousands of dollars' worth of items from off-price retailers simply because they had the bright yellow clearance tags on them. The isolation I felt during those months only intensified my emotional grief. I justified purchasing countless decorative pillows, charcuterie boards, wall mirrors, and shoes thinking that these items could somehow fill the void created by social distancing and lack of interaction. Each purchase offered a brief high, a distraction from the loneliness, but it ultimately left me feeling even emptier.

Then came buyer's remorse. Compulsive shopping can lead to feelings of guilt and regret, creating a vicious cycle where shopping becomes a temporary escape from emotional pain. Instead of confronting underlying issues, these patterned behaviors mask them, and that's why it's crucial to recognize the complexities of modern addictions. While they may seem less severe than substance abuse, their emotional and psychological impacts can still be profound, affecting not just individuals but also their relationships and overall well-being.

Ultimately, understanding these patterns in our behavior can empower us to seek healthier coping mechanisms and address the root causes of our distress.

Embracing a Holistic Approach

As I reflect on my journey, I've come to realize something incredibly important: the truths about our childhood are deeply embedded in our bodies, no matter how hard we try to suppress them. Dr. Bessel van der Kolk (2014) emphasizes this connection, stating that "the body keeps the score" and that traumatic experiences can become ingrained in our physical selves, impacting our mental and emotional well-being. I know medication can feel like a lifeline, offering temporary relief, but it often misses the deeper issues that linger beneath the surface. Trust me when I say that unless we confront those hidden pains and truly begin to heal, they will continue to haunt us. You might feel okay for months or even years, but eventually those unresolved feelings will catch up to you. Please don't ignore this. It's what led me to seek out alternative solutions that addressed my whole being and it's made all the difference.

Having been off antidepressants for almost 10 months, I discovered that methods such as journaling, meditation, and breathing exercises were significantly more effective when managing my mental health. Incorporating emotional freedom techniques (EFT)—tapping and exploring supplements— also played a role in enhancing my well-being. This made it clear to me: medication is only one component of a broader array of resources to improve mental health.

This experience highlighted the importance of finding a healthcare provider who offers a variety of treatment options. Compassionate care goes beyond just prescribing medication; it involves a personalized approach that takes your unique experiences into account. Combining different methods— whether conventional or alternative—can lead to a more tailored and effective path to healing.

Many of us feel frustrated by the repetitive cycle of doctor visits, where the same prescriptions are handed out without a deeper exploration of our symptoms. This pattern of temporary relief often leads us to seek a more comprehensive approach. And through my own experience, the integration of Internal Family Systems (IFS) theory provided a valuable new perspective.

In our recent discussions, we examined how Internal Family Systems (IFS) provide a unique perspective that transcends the traditional emphasis on symptoms and diagnoses. Instead of primarily seeing ourselves through anxiety, self-criticism, or other challenges, IFS suggests that we view these as components of a broader, interconnected system within us. Our past experiences have influenced aspects of us that don't define our whole identity—they've evolved as a means of self-protection, even if they occasionally cause conflict or discomfort.

The core of IFS is really about recognizing and embracing these different parts with empathy instead of criticism. By accepting challenges, we work with them, which promotes healing. Your inner experiences, regardless of how tough they may be, are completely valid. When you approach them with kindness, it opens up opportunities for significant change, resulting in a more cohesive and empowered sense of self.

When paired with medication and additional supportive practices, IFS provides a deeper insight into mental health. Medication can definitely be a useful resource, but it's just one part of a bigger approach. A well-rounded approach that incorporates empathy for the inner self while acknowledging the constraints of a strictly scientific perspective can result in deeper and more significant healing. Remember, you're not alone in this; exploring various methods and seeking assistance can significantly transform your situation.

Interactive Exercise: Building Your Support Network

Draw a visual map of your support network. Place yourself at the center and connect to those who uplift and support you—friends, family, colleagues, and online communities. Look at how these connections help you and identify any gaps. If some relationships feel like dead leaves cluttering your space, give yourself permission to gently prune them and make room for fresh, vibrant connections.

Celebrate every bit of progress, like tending to your inner garden—even if it sometimes feels like you're battling a jungle of emotions! Remember, just as plants need sunlight, you need moments of self-care and encouragement. Keep your support network blooming with love and joy and enjoy every burst of growth along the way. Your dedication to creating this nurturing environment shows just how amazing and resilient you are. Keep blooming and shining!

Support Network Reflection:

- Who are the people you turn to for support?
- How do they help you feel more balanced and less overwhelmed?
- Are there any new relationships you'd like to cultivate or existing ones you'd like to strengthen?

Building a safe, non-judgmental space is all about being gentle with yourself and making thoughtful choices. By fostering this environment you'll find it easier to open up and heal, knowing you're supported every step of the way.

Reach Out Challenge

I have a challenge for you this week: reach out to someone who makes you feel supported. Whether it's sending a heartfelt text, giving them a call, arranging a coffee date, or connecting through an online community, take a moment to express your gratitude. Acknowledge those who have been there for you and explore ways to strengthen these connections. Pay attention to how sharing your load, even in small ways, affects your sense of connection and support. Document your experience and reflect on the impact these interactions have on your feelings of belonging and encouragement. Remember, there are many people rooting for you and cheering you on.

CHAPTER 11

Setting Boundaries with Love

Identifying Your Personal Boundary Needs

"The Oxygen Mask"

Julie sat quietly at the kitchen table, her coffee growing cold as the familiar chaos of the morning swirled around her. Her three children were getting ready for school, each calling out for her attention in different ways—missing shoes, an unfinished science project, and the last-minute snack requests. She loved her children fiercely, but lately, she had found herself feeling depleted, like she was running on empty.

It wasn't always like this. She had once been full of energy, juggling all the tasks with grace. But something had shifted. The constant demands, the endless responsibilities—she didn't realize how much they were draining her until exhaustion became her norm. She found herself snapping at her kids over small things, resenting her husband for not noticing her fatigue, and barely recognizing the woman staring back at her in the mirror.

One afternoon, after yet another day of feeling spread too thinly, Julie sat down with her journal. As she wrote, a phrase came to mind: "Secure your own oxygen mask first." She remembered the safety instructions from her last flight, telling passengers to put on their own oxygen mask before helping others. It hit her like a revelation. She had been so focused on taking care of everyone else that she had forgotten to take care of herself.

Her mind wandered to the idea of boundaries—something she had brushed off in the past. Boundaries felt selfish, like saying "no" would somehow make her less of a good mother. But now she was beginning to understand that boundaries weren't about keeping people out; they were about making space for her own well-being. They were about recognizing her worth and creating a safe space where she could truly flourish.

She thought about the times she had stayed up late to finish laundry or said "yes" to things she didn't have the energy for, only to end up frustrated and burnt out. These moments weren't just minor annoyances—they were signs that she had been ignoring her own needs. Her sense of self had become tangled up in the expectations of everyone around her, leaving little room for who she truly was.

Over the next few weeks, Julie began to make small changes. She started with simple things—like taking 10 minutes in the morning to drink her coffee in peace, setting boundaries around her time, and learning to say "no" when she needed to. At first, it felt uncomfortable, even guilt-inducing, but soon, she began to notice a shift.

She wasn't just surviving the day anymore; she was finding moments to breathe. She found herself being more patient with her kids, more present with her husband, and even more connected with herself. Instead of feeling drained by the endless to-do lists, she felt a renewed sense of clarity and purpose. By tending to her own "oxygen mask," she was able to show up as the mother she wanted to be—more grounded, more loving, and more whole.

The more Julie focused on her boundaries the more she realized they weren't walls to keep people out. Instead, they were the foundation for stronger, healthier relationships. With her newfound energy, she could listen more intently to her children, empathize with their struggles, and still have enough left over for herself.

In the end, Julie learned that boundaries weren't about isolation; they were about connection. They were about creating space to truly thrive, both as a mother and as a woman. And in doing so, she discovered that by taking care of herself, she could take better care of the ones she loved.

Keep in mind that establishing and upholding boundaries is a process and it's perfectly fine to approach it gradually. Engaging in practices such as breathwork and journaling can be incredibly beneficial—breathwork keeps you centered and journaling provides a space to contemplate your needs and pinpoint areas that may require change. Moreover, somatic therapy can assist in reestablishing a connection with your body's reactions to stress and trauma, helping to release tension that has accumulated from past experiences. Being more in tune with your body's signals can help lower stress and anxiety, which in turn supports healing and emotional balance (National Center for Complementary and Integrative Health [NCCIH], 2024). These practices together help you move toward healthier and more balanced relationships.

Above all, approach this journey with compassion. Boundaries are not about distancing yourself from others—they're about creating a space where you can peacefully thrive and love can grow.

Understanding the Importance of Boundaries in Healing

Establishing boundaries is incredibly important, especially for mothers dealing with past traumas. Think of boundaries as emotional and psychological shields that help you maintain balance and well-being. For mothers, who often find themselves busy giving and nurturing, setting these boundaries becomes even more crucial. Not only is this beneficial for you as a mom but it also models self-respect and healthy emotional regulation for your children.

Trauma can alter with our sense of self-care versus self-sacrifice. Without clear boundaries, old wounds pop up and affect our mental health and relationships with our kids and partners. Setting clear but loving limits lets moms create a safe space for themselves while also providing stability for their families.

Boundaries aren't just about saying "no" or drawing lines; they're about taking back control and making sure your needs are met without feeling guilty. This is especially important if you've had trauma as it gives you a sense of agency that might have been lost before. By setting boundaries with love you balance caring for yourself while caring for others.

Recognizing the Impact of Past Traumas on Your Present

Understanding how the baggage you carry affects you is a crucial step in setting healthy boundaries, especially on your healing journey. Past traumas can subtly shape how we act and react today, impacting our interactions with our children, spouses, and even ourselves.

By now, you've likely recognized that some of your triggers or reactions stem from unresolved issues. For instance, a mother who felt neglected as a child might grapple with feelings of inadequacy or fear of abandonment. These emotions can lead her to overcompensate by being overly permissive or overly protective, confusing supportive parenting with enabling unhealthy behavior—something we explored in Chapter 4.

Self-awareness is key on this journey. It involves compassionately exploring your life story and acknowledging how your past has shaped your present. This awareness empowers you to set boundaries with love and self-respect, fostering healthier relationships and creating a supportive, harmonious environment for your family.

Remember, this process is about growth. Treat yourself with the same kindness you offer others as you navigate these changes. Self-awareness is central to lasting, positive transformation—a recurring theme throughout this book for a reason.

Communicating Boundaries with Compassion and Clarity

Communicating boundaries with compassion and clarity is crucial, especially for moms juggling their own healing alongside family life. Picture this: you're in the middle of a busy day, pulled in multiple directions, and you feel that familiar pang of overwhelm rising. That's when you realize—this is your body telling you something important. It's a signal that your needs or limits are being stretched.

Understanding these signals is the first step in setting boundaries, not just for your well-being but also for nurturing healthier relationships. When you tune in to these feelings, you create space to pause, reflect, and ask yourself: *What do I need right now?* This kind of self-awareness lets you approach conversations with loved ones from a place of empathy and calm, making boundary-setting a more compassionate, natural process.

In Internal Family Systems (IFS), boundary-setting involves engaging with different parts of you—exiles, managers, and firefighters. Each part has its own emotional responses and perspectives and addressing them with empathy can make these conversations more supportive and understanding.

Understanding and Engaging Your Parts:

Exiles: These are the parts of you that hold deep emotional pain and vulnerability. When setting boundaries, approach these parts with tenderness. For example, if you're feeling overwhelmed, instead of saying, "You never help with the kids," which may unintentionally hurt these vulnerable parts, try saying, "I'm feeling quite overwhelmed with the bedtime routine. I would really appreciate your help to ease the load. Can we work out a schedule that allows me some downtime?" This way, you're acknowledging their needs while inviting support.

Managers: These parts of you strive to maintain control and order but can sometimes feel stressed or pressured when boundaries aren't clear. Instead of saying, "You always forget your chores," which might feel like a criticism, try expressing, "I'm feeling stressed when chores pile up. Could we create a list together to keep track of what needs to be done?" This approach supports both your needs and theirs, fostering cooperation.

Firefighters: These parts react quickly to avoid emotional discomfort and may become defensive when boundaries are discussed. Rather than saying, "You keep canceling our plans," which might trigger guilt or defensiveness, consider, "I feel disappointed when our plans fall through. Can we find a time that works better for both of us to catch up?" This approach acknowledges your feelings while opening the door to a constructive solution.

Applying Emotional Granularity and Emotional Intelligence:

Emotional Granularity

Being specific about your feelings and needs is super important when it comes to effective communication. Instead of saying something vague like, "I need more help," try being more precise: "I need assistance with the evening routine on weekdays so I can have some quiet time to recharge." This kind of clarity not only helps others understand exactly what you're asking for but also highlights why it's important to you. By clearly expressing your needs, you give others the chance to respond in a meaningful way, which can lead to better support. Research shows that practicing emotional granularity—being able to identify and articulate nuanced emotions—can actually lower anxiety and depression as it helps you develop better coping strategies and stronger connections with others.

Emotional Intelligence (EQ)

Emotional intelligence (EQ) is all about being aware of your own emotions and understanding how they impact those around you. This awareness is key for building healthy relationships. When you approach conversations, it's crucial to do so with empathy and a willingness to listen. For example, while you're sharing your needs, make sure to also consider the other person's perspective and feelings. This kind of balance helps create a dialogue that's respectful and supportive. Studies have shown that having high emotional intelligence can lead to more effective communication, conflict resolution, and collaboration. By practicing active listening—where you not only hear what someone is saying but also pick up on their underlying emotions—you can build a deeper connection that fosters trust and mutual respect.

Quick Recap: Emotional Granularity vs. Emotional Intelligence

Emotional Granularity is all about the ability to pinpoint and articulate specific emotions and needs. It helps you communicate clearly, allowing others to understand exactly what you require and why it matters.

Emotional Intelligence (EQ) encompasses a broader skill set, including self-awareness and empathy. It's about understanding your own emotions and how they affect those around you, fostering healthier interactions and deeper connections.

In short, emotional granularity helps you express yourself while emotional intelligence helps you navigate and respond to the emotions of others.

Fostering Mutual Respect and Empathy:

When you show empathy by recognizing and validating the other person's feelings while also expressing your own needs, you create a foundation of mutual respect. This kind of open communication fosters an atmosphere where everyone feels heard and valued. Setting boundaries becomes less about drawing lines and more about creating a balanced space where everyone's needs are acknowledged. It's this balance that strengthens relationships and builds deeper understanding.

Integrating IFS insights into these conversations allows you to express your needs with clarity while also cultivating a sense of care and connection. In this way, setting boundaries not only supports your healing but also fosters more compassionate, healthier relationships with those around you.

Self-Care Practices to Support Ongoing Healing and Boundary Setting

Self-care is a vital part of setting boundaries, particularly for mothers or any individual healing from trauma. It's not about occasional treats but about consistent practices that nurture your mental and emotional well-being. Start by understanding your needs, triggers, and limits to set boundaries that respect both you and others.

By now you're familiar with incorporating mindfulness practices regularly, which can help you stay present and in tune with yourself. Seeking support from communities or professionals, like therapy or support groups, can provide validation and encouragement. Physical self-care—such as exercise, balanced nutrition, and adequate rest and sleep—also plays a huge role in mental health, making it easier to manage stress and make clear boundary decisions.

Lastly, practice self-compassion. The journey through trauma is rarely straightforward and setbacks are a natural part of the process. As I write this book, I want to be clear that I am definitely not speaking from a place of perfection. My insights come from ongoing growth and shared experiences, not from a state of complete resolution. We're all healing and growing together, navigating this path side by side, and every step you take is a powerful move forward.

Take a moment to truly celebrate the progress you've made, no matter how small it may feel. Each step you take, even the simplest ones, holds the potential for profound transformation. It's important to remember that being kind to yourself during the tough times isn't just a nice idea; it's an act of courage. These moments of self-kindness build resilience and strengthen your ability to maintain healthy boundaries, allowing you to protect not just yourself but also your loved ones.

In the upcoming chapters, we'll explore how self-compassion can be a guiding light on your path to long-term well-being. As mothers, we often carry the weight of our past traumas and it can be challenging to extend grace to ourselves. But embracing self-compassion is a reflection of your strength and dedication to healing. It's about acknowledging that you've been through a lot and giving yourself permission to feel, to grieve, and to grow.

Remember, it's okay to recognize the struggles you face—they're part of your journey, not a sign of weakness. By honoring your experiences and treating yourself with the kindness you so readily offer to others, you empower yourself to move forward. You're not just surviving; you're actively choosing to thrive, and that is remarkable proof of your fortitude and commitment to healing.

"Abs, Grief & Implants"

In January 2015, I began what I thought would be the ultimate test of my strength—a 12-week bodybuilding transformation program. I threw myself into it, determined to gain control over my body. My days were consumed by eating, training, and sleeping. I worked out twice a day, six days a week, for hours on end, pushing myself to the limit. By the end of it, I was proud of the physical results—lean, with visible abs, and a body fat percentage under 10%. It felt like I had reached a peak, a moment of triumph.

But shortly after, everything changed. My husband and I found out we were expecting a baby, and for a brief moment, joy filled my world. That joy was shattered when my first sonogram revealed no heartbeat. I was devastated. I blamed myself—blamed my body—for not being able to hold on to our baby. I couldn't shake the belief that my extreme training had somehow contributed to this loss. It was my first miscarriage and I didn't know how to process the grief. Instead, I carried it deep inside, convinced that something was wrong with me, with my body.

As I struggled to cope with the heartbreak, I made a decision that I thought would help me reclaim some sense of control. Later that year, I underwent breast augmentation, telling myself that I didn't want more children. I was terrified of facing another loss, another heartache. But the surgery didn't bring the relief I had hoped for. Instead, it compounded my pain. A few days after the procedure, I developed complications—my left breast was bruised, swollen, and no longer symmetrical. What I thought would boost my confidence only deepened my insecurities. I became more self-conscious, constantly reminded that I had tried to "fix" something on the outside while the inside was still broken.

Looking back, I realize now how deeply intertwined my body image, my grief, and my unresolved traumas were. The miscarriage, the surgery, the emotional wounds—they were all pieces of a larger puzzle I was trying to put together. I thought changing my body would help me heal, but it only highlighted the pain I hadn't yet addressed.

This journey has shown me how often we try to control or 'fix' our physical selves when our emotional wounds remain untreated. I've learned that true healing doesn't come from changing how we look—it comes from acknowledging and working through the pain we carry inside.

If you're reading this and you've felt the weight of unresolved trauma, please know you're not alone. The path to healing is not easy, but it doesn't have to be walked alone.

CHAPTER 12

Embracing and Transforming Shame, Guilt, and Anger

Acknowledging Your Journey

As we near the end of this book, it's essential to recognize and celebrate the progress you've made. Consider the moments you've taken to reflect on your feelings or the times you've chosen to respond to your children with understanding instead of frustration. These steps signify your commitment to personal growth. This chapter builds upon the foundation you've established, offering practical tools and compassionate insights to help you navigate these complex emotions with confidence and gentleness. Remember, the journey continues and you are equipped with the skills to handle these emotions effectively.

Understanding Shame

Shame is a deep-seated feeling that whispers to you that there is something fundamentally wrong with who you are. Unlike guilt, which focuses on specific actions, shame reflects the self—evoking feelings of unworthiness, flaw, or inadequacy. This emotion often surfaces in moments when you perceive yourself as failing to meet personal or societal expectations, leaving you with a heavy heart and a profound sense of isolation. You may find yourself wondering if you truly belong, feeling as if you are constantly falling short.

The Roots of Shame

Shame frequently has its origins in early events that affect your self-image. Consider moments when a disapproving look or harsh words from a parent made you doubt your value. In my own cultural upbringing, violations I experienced were rarely addressed. The concept of therapy was nonexistent and conversations about feelings were dismissed and brushed under the rug. This lack of recognition produced a gap of unacknowledged anguish that had a significant impact on my self-image. According to Brené Brown (2012), shame is a universal feeling that has a significant impact on our sense of belonging and self-worth, often causing us to accept the assumption that our value is conditional. Recognizing these early effects is critical to understanding how they still affect our behaviors and perceptions now.

The Impact of Shame on Other Emotions

Shame looms large over other emotions, often overlapping with guilt and anger. For example, after committing a mistake, you may experience a rush of shame, followed by remorse for your actions or anger against yourself. This emotional cycle might make you feel trapped since shame impairs your capacity to react positively. Understanding how shame drives these feelings allows you to start unraveling the layers and addressing them more effectively.

Acknowledging your shame is the first step toward healing. Recognizing the effect might help you replace self-judgment with compassion and empathy. Embracing this process helps transform shame and builds resilience as you grow and heal.

Naming the Shame

As you develop the muscle to now identify and recognize the voice of shame, you can stop it before it spirals into self destructive criticisms and replace them with self-affirming truths. The following exercise is a series of questions that holds key to sources of your shame.

Were you made to feel in charge of the mental health or emotional condition of another person?

Were you compared unfavorably to other kids?

Did you ever feel that, despite your best efforts, you were not good enough?

Did anyone abandon you?

Have you ever been told that you're not worthy of success or happiness?

Did you have to conceal or repress aspects of yourself in order to be accepted?

Did somebody ever give you the impression that you were always at fault, regardless of the circumstances?

Were you neglected?

Did your feelings, actions, or decisions cause you to feel ashamed?

In what ways were you humiliated, belittled, or demeaned?

Has someone ever minimized or discounted your suffering?

Were you made to feel unwanted? Unacceptable? Useless?

Have you ever been manipulated or controlled in a manner that caused you to question your value?

Were you made to feel wrong, bad, or stupid?

Were you taunted or teased by other kids?

Did you experience exclusion or rejection from peer or family groups?

Were you abused, physically, verbally, or sexually?

It takes courage and healing to name what shames us, and it can lighten the burden of silence and secrecy. When we put words to our shame, we take away its power and open the door to self-compassion and growth. It's a way of saying, "This doesn't define me," and allows us to connect with others who can offer empathy and understanding.

Identifying your shame is a significant step in taking back your narrative and discovering strength in your vulnerability. You're not the only one who feels shame; everyone does. You deserve the comfort and healing that come with knowing that you can do this.

Exploring Guilt

Guilt arises when you feel you have done something wrong or failed to meet certain standards. Unlike shame, which envelops the self in a cloud of unworthiness, guilt focuses on specific actions or behaviors. It often brings with it a wave of remorse and a deep desire to make amends. You might find yourself revisiting moments when you felt you let someone down—perhaps recalling a time when you missed an important event in your child's life or neglected a promise to a loved one. For those carrying unresolved trauma, these moments can feel even heavier as past wounds amplify the emotional stakes of your present actions.

The Roots of Guilt

Your beliefs and cultural standards intimately link to guilt, which often stems from early events that stay with you. Imagine you chose to favor work over your child's school play only to experience a knot in your gut as you recollect their disappointed expression. These memories remain, creating a profound sense of regret that may affect your everyday life.

For mothers who are still struggling with unresolved trauma this psychological tug-of-war may be particularly intense. Past wounds may affect your perception of right and wrong, turning daily actions into moral dilemmas. Consider navigating a situation where you had to say "no" to a friend in need. Instead of feeling justified, self-doubt might haunt you, replaying the scenario in your mind and questioning your motives.

When your actions contradict your underlying convictions or you fail to meet the high standards you set for yourself, shame may become a regular companion. It whispers reminders of what you regard as failures, leading you to rethink decisions with a sorrowful spirit. Perhaps you feel guilty when you spend time for yourself, believing that you should constantly prioritize others. This never-ending pattern might make you feel stuck, as if you're carrying a weight that becomes heavier with each passing day.

Recognizing this pattern is the first step toward understanding and healing. By identifying the origins of your guilt you can begin to differentiate between emotions that are a reflection of your past and those that are authentic to your beliefs. This awareness can pave the way for self-compassion and the ability to forgive yourself for being human.

Gender Perspectives on Guilt

It's also important to consider gender perspectives in understanding guilt. Research indicates that women often report higher levels of guilt than men, influenced by societal expectations and gender roles. Women are frequently socialized to prioritize relationships and caregiving, leading to feelings of guilt when they perceive they have let others down. This societal conditioning can amplify feelings of inadequacy, making it harder to forgive yourself for perceived shortcomings. As a mother, you might find yourself feeling guilty for not being the perfect parent, reflecting on how your upbringing and cultural context have shaped these expectations.

Guilt's Connection to Shame and Anger

Guilt frequently follows shame, especially for those with unresolved trauma. This is because guilt often relates to specific actions rooted in a deeper sense of inadequacy. For example, if you find yourself snapping at your child in a moment of frustration, the guilt that follows may be compounded by feelings of shame tied to your own past experiences. This interplay intensifies your emotional struggle, making it hard to separate past hurts from present actions.

Additionally, unresolved guilt can fester and contribute to feelings of anger—either directed at yourself for perceived failures or toward others who may have influenced your sense of inadequacy. Understanding this connection can illuminate how trauma informs your emotional landscape, helping you navigate your feelings more effectively.

Managing Anger

Anger is a natural emotional response to perceived wrongs or injustices. It can manifest outwardly, like a shout or a heated argument, or inwardly, causing a storm of frustration within. Often, it arises when you feel your needs or boundaries have been violated. When a boundary is crossed, you might feel adrenaline coursing through your body, igniting a fight-or-flight response. It's essential to recognize that anger can be a secondary emotion, frequently triggered by deeper feelings of shame or guilt. By understanding this dynamic, you can begin to address your anger in a healthier way.

The Roots of Anger

Anger often emerges when you feel unjustly treated or threatened. Take a moment to reflect on a situation where your values were disrespected. How did that anger manifest? Perhaps you felt a tightening in your chest, a rush of heat in your face, or a clenched jaw. These physical sensations are your body's way of signaling that something needs your attention.

Furthermore, rage might be a result of unresolved guilt or shame, so it's important to identify what's driving the emotions you are experiencing. Many women who have unresolved trauma may experience an internal struggle that blurs the distinction between their current problems and past experiences. Even though anger may seem overwhelming, understanding it as a signal of other emotions present can be empowering.

Recent research highlights that anger serves a dual role. On one hand, it acts as an inward signal indicating a need to confront obstacles or unpleasant situations, motivating you to seek change. On the other hand, anger is an outwardly directed communicative signal, establishing boundaries and addressing conflicts within relationships. By exploring these underlying emotions you can transform anger from a reactive force into a constructive one that drives positive change, allowing you to advocate for your needs while fostering healthier connections with others.

Healthy Outlets for Anger

Managing anger effectively involves finding constructive ways to express and channel it. Consider these strategies:

1. **Mindfulness**: Cultivate the practice of being present with your emotions. Allow your anger to surface without judgment. Acknowledge its presence without letting it control you, creating space for reflection and understanding.

2. **Physical Exercise**: Engage in activities that release built-up tension, such as brisk walking, gym workouts, or dancing. Physical activity alleviates stress and boosts endorphins, improving your mood.

3. **Assertive Communication**: Express your feelings and needs clearly and respectfully to prevent escalation. Use "I" statements, like, "I feel hurt when my opinions are dismissed," to foster understanding and ensure your voice is heard.

4. **Creative Outlets**: Channel your anger into creative activities—writing, painting, or playing music. These outlets allow for constructive emotional expression and foster healing.

5. **Seeking Support**: Reach out to friends, family, or a therapist. Discussing your feelings can provide perspective and help you develop healthier coping strategies.

Strategies for Transforming These Emotions

Processing and Releasing Shame and Guilt

To address shame and guilt, consider the following:

- **Self-Compassion**: Treat yourself with the kindness you would offer a friend. When you stumble, envision giving yourself a comforting hug. Kristin Neff (2011) emphasizes that self-compassion fosters resilience and emotional well-being.
- **Cognitive Restructuring**: Challenge negative beliefs about yourself. When self-doubt arises, replace it with affirmations of your worth and capability. Visualize negative thoughts as clouds drifting away as you acknowledge them.
- **Forgiveness Practices**: Work on forgiving yourself for past mistakes. Understand that forgiveness is a process and letting go of self-blame can lead to healing.

Managing Anger Constructively

In addition to the techniques mentioned, try these approaches:

- **Reflective Practices**: Use journaling or meditation to explore the sources of your anger and its connections to other emotions. Picture yourself writing down your feelings, transforming the weight of your anger into clarity on the page.
- **Boundaries and Assertiveness**: Establish and maintain clear boundaries to protect your emotional well-being. Communicate assertively to address conflicts and prevent anger from festering.

Connecting with Your Inner Self

Engaging with your inner self involves:

- **Self-Reflection**: Take time to explore your emotional landscape. Reflect on how shame, guilt, and anger influence your behavior and relationships. Consider pausing to check in with yourself—what do you feel?
- **Meditation and Journaling**: Use these tools to engage with your emotions and gain insights into your experiences. They can help you integrate and understand different aspects of your emotional self.

Embracing Your Ongoing Journey

As you integrate these practices into your life, remember to approach yourself with the same kindness and patience you've cultivated throughout this book. The tools and insights you've gained are meant to empower you, offering a supportive framework for navigating and transforming these emotions. Trust in your growth, honor your journey, and continue to embrace the path of self-discovery with confidence and compassion. Your journey of emotional understanding and self-empowerment is ongoing and you are well-equipped to continue this path with grace and strength.

"Is this what peace feels like?"

After the birth of my fifth child, I found myself in a place I had never expected—grappling with the physical and emotional manifestations of trauma. My life had always been centered on health and wellness. I maintained a colorful, nutritious diet, exercised regularly, and had always prided myself on staying fit. But just weeks before my daughter's arrival, everything changed when I slipped and fell in a restaurant. The impact was sudden and jarring, but I dismissed it as a minor accident, not realizing the significance it would soon have on my health.

Three days after giving birth, I was rushed back to the hospital, diagnosed with postpartum preeclampsia. My blood pressure had surged to a dangerous 100/200, signaling something far deeper unraveling within me. That same year, I was diagnosed with diverticulitis. My once strong, resilient body now felt foreign. My blood pressure was erratic and I developed rashes on my face and body along with inflamed joints, blurred vision, and dramatic weight fluctuations. My body seemed to be in overdrive, betraying me despite how devoted and committed I was to wellness.

I also began suffering from debilitating migraines, which had followed me throughout my life, dating back to my teenage years. One particularly severe episode occurred when my firstborn was five months old. Every time I sat up, it felt like my head was being crushed from within. Lying down provided temporary relief, but after five long days, two ER visits, and a spinal tap that worsened the pain the doctors discovered a cerebrospinal fluid leak. A blood patch procedure brought almost immediate relief, as if a weight had been lifted. But, soon, other challenges emerged.

In the background of all this was my lifelong struggle with anxiety and depression. Since my teenage years, I had been managing it quietly, a subscriber to antidepressants, with Celexa serving as my hidden companion. After my fifth child, I was prescribed Lexapro for what was termed "baby blues," but I knew it wasn't just that. The medication helped me get through the day, but I couldn't shake the feeling that there was something deeper I needed to address.

Then, in September 2022, things took a sharp turn. I had been battling a lingering headache and a general sense of malaise throughout the day. That evening, while watching a documentary on Jeffrey Dahmer, the unease intensified. I brushed it off, thinking it was just the unsettling nature of the show. But later that night, something shifted dramatically. I woke up in an ambulance, disoriented and vomiting, with no clear memory of what had happened. After a series of tests, I was told it was a panic attack. From that night onward, my health took a sudden and alarming dive, leaving me wondering if something deeper had been triggered.

My usual 6:00 a.m. CrossFit routines were replaced by days where I could sleep for up to 16 hours. Even climbing the stairs felt like a monumental task. I began experiencing frequent palpitations—sudden, racing heartbeats that left me feeling uneasy and out of breath. I was prescribed an inhaler for the shortness of breath, but nothing seemed to alleviate the exhaustion and rapid decline I was experiencing. I barely recognized myself anymore.

Determined to get answers, I did my own research and sought out consultations. Breast implant illness came up in conversations and the symptoms I read about eerily mirrored my own. I was certain I had finally found the answer. I began perusing breast implant illness communities, reading stories from women whose experiences matched mine almost exactly. I was certain this was what was wrong with me. I became determined to have the implants removed, even though it would cost twice as much as I had originally paid, and since it wasn't considered a medical necessity, insurance wouldn't cover it. It felt like everything finally made sense. But as time went on, my health continued to fluctuate—some days were better while others were much worse. I kept searching, still determined to find clarity.

Over the years, I saw countless specialists—every "-ologist" you can name—and underwent numerous tests, blood work, and scans, all of which showed that I was perfectly fine. The results left me baffled. My symptoms were real, yet I was told there was nothing wrong. This only deepened my frustration and left me in limbo, searching for any diagnosis that could explain what was happening to me.

Then came a flicker of hope. One test revealed an anomaly in my **RNA** polymerase iii (ribonucleic acid), a molecule essential for coding, decoding, regulation, and expression of genes, which was linked to my **ANA** (antinuclear antibodies)—a type of autoantibody often present in autoimmune disorder such as systemic sclerosis. *This must be it,* I thought. The shortness of breath, the fatigue; all of it. For the first time in a long while, I felt a sense of validation. I would have gladly accepted any diagnosis just to have an explanation, but even this answer didn't provide the clarity I craved.

Throughout this period, anxiety continued to overshadow everything. It wasn't just the physical symptoms; it was the constant sense of dread that I couldn't escape. Panic attacks would strike unexpectedly, turning routine moments into overwhelming ones. Driving, particularly on the freeway, became a source of debilitating fear. Unless absolutely necessary, I avoided it altogether.

In January 2024, I finally did something that had terrified me for years—I saw my father for the first time in 24 years. For so long, the thought of facing him felt like cowardice, like I wasn't brave enough to confront the past. I didn't know what to expect when we met, but now, as I sit here writing this, I realize something I never anticipated: since that day, my body feels different. The symptoms that had plagued me for so long—aches, anxiety, that constant, unshakable tension—they've started to ease. My health, which used to be a storm, now feels calmer, like something deep within me has settled. Maybe this is what healing looks like.

I keep coming back to that word—healing. Maybe this is what my body has been waiting for all along: peace.

Looking back, I wonder if that fall in the restaurant—the sharp jolt—stirred something much deeper than I realized. It wasn't just a physical accident; it felt like it cracked open years of buried trauma. Trauma I had thought I could ignore. But after that fall, everything I had buried seemed to rise to the surface. The physical pain, the emotional mess, the anxiety and depression—it all came rushing back, along with memories I'd tried hard to suppress. The sexual violations I experienced as a child, the hurt, fear, shame, anger, guilt, confusion—all the things I hadn't fully processed.

It took me years to realize that trauma doesn't just live in our minds; it buries itself deep inside our bodies. Every chest pain, every headache, every flare-up—those weren't just symptoms; they were sirens. My body was asking me to stop running, to stop pretending I could heal without confronting the darkness I had tucked away.

And maybe, just maybe, after all these years, I'm finally beginning to understand. Healing isn't about erasing the pain or forgetting the past. It's about confronting it—head-on. It's about letting it rise to the surface, facing it with honesty and vulnerability, and confronting it rather than running from it.

Maybe this is what peace feels like.

CHAPTER 13

Embracing Self-Compassion

Understanding the Connection between Safety and Healing

Let's start by talking about something fundamental—safety. Feeling safe, especially in our own bodies, is crucial for healing. When we're dealing with trauma or everyday stress, our bodies can tense up, creating a barrier that blocks emotional expression. This tension signals that something isn't right and that we're not feeling entirely safe.

Mothers may experience this more intensely due to the constant demands and societal norms that disregard our needs. However, healing begins when we are comfortable with who we are. We may release the knots of tension that have accumulated over time by respecting our feelings rather than repressing them. These simple practices help support us in reestablishing our connection to our body and emotions.

One reason mothers often struggle to feel safe in their bodies is somatic memory—the body's ability to store and recall traumatic experiences through physical sensations, even when the conscious mind has forgotten them. The nervous system stores trauma, whether from past experiences or the pressures of motherhood, resulting in ongoing physical discomfort that mirrors unresolved emotions. This stored trauma can manifest as chronic tension, pain, or anxiety.

From the moment we learn we're expecting, our bodies and identities undergo profound changes, leaving us feeling disconnected from our former selves. These transformations are not just physical; they also significantly affect our emotional and mental well-being. Society's expectations for mothers to be flawless, selfless caregivers often make it challenging to prioritize personal needs, leading to emotional strain that physically manifests as tension, anxiety, and guilt. Acknowledging these challenges is the first step toward healing, allowing us to reconnect with our true selves and become the mothers we aspire to be.

Emotional suppression further complicates our well-being. When we bury our feelings, our bodies bear the burden, storing unprocessed stress and trauma in the nervous system, which manages our stress responses. This cycle of emotional neglect intensifies until our bodies rebel, signaling that something needs attention. Physical symptoms like tightness in the chest or knots in the stomach are not merely stress responses; they indicate unresolved emotional issues.

Unresolved emotional stress often leads to physical manifestations for many mothers, including chronic pain, tension in the neck, back, or shoulders, and anxiety. Everyday triggers, such as the sound of a crying child or a specific smell, can evoke physiological reactions, serving as signals that unresolved trauma remains. Over time, these repressed emotions can lead to panic attacks or anxiety, often associated with the pain the body continues to carry.

Cultivating Safety within You and Your Body

To begin the healing process, start by acknowledging and validating your emotions. Mindfulness and meditation can help you stay present and recognize the body's signals. This brings us to *somatic awareness*—the practice of tuning into your body's physical sensations, where unresolved emotional pain often resides.

For years, I struggled to understand why, during yoga classes, I would find myself unexpectedly crying, especially at the end of sessions or after certain poses. At the time, I couldn't make sense of it—there was no conscious reason for the tears. It was only later that I realized my body had been holding on to unresolved trauma and pain, emotions that I had buried deep and were still stored in the fibers of my being. Yoga, with its focus on breath and movement, had opened a pathway for those emotions to surface, offering an outlet for my body to release what my mind had long suppressed.

This experience is not uncommon and highlights how the body holds on to trauma. Trauma, even when mentally suppressed, is often stored in the body's tissues, muscles, and nervous system. The release of emotions during physical activities like yoga occurs because movement helps unlock these stored memories. Neuroscience supports this as well—when we engage in practices like yoga or bodywork, it stimulates the vagus nerve, which is integral to the parasympathetic nervous system responsible for calming the body. This nerve, when activated through breathwork or physical movement, helps the body process and release stored emotions, sometimes leading to crying or emotional surges.

Dr. Peter Levine, founder of Somatic Experiencing, emphasizes this connection between the body and emotional healing, stating, "The sensations in our body provide us with an innate wisdom that is often overlooked." By engaging in somatic awareness—being mindful of what your body is telling you—you can identify when you're holding on to stress and trauma. As you become more attuned to your body, emotional releases like mine during yoga make more sense: they are part of the healing process, allowing us to let go of what's been too painful to confront at the time and to foster emotional safety and embrace self-compassion, particularly if you tend to be self-critical. This mindset helps create a safe internal environment for healing. Prioritize self-care activities that deepen your connection with your body, such as relaxation, bodywork, or even simple movements like stretching. These activities encourage the release of stored tension and trauma, creating space for emotional healing.

Additionally, create a comforting space in your home where you can retreat when feeling overwhelmed. Fill it with calming items, such as pillows or essential oils, and use it for journaling, breathwork, or meditation. This can become your sanctuary for processing emotions. As you work through these practices, you may find that moments of release, like the ones I experienced in yoga, become less frightening and more welcome as signs of healing.

Self-Compassion and Body Acceptance

Please allow me to share something very personal and meaningful. As I look back on my journey I realize that I once held a belief that pre-mom bodies represented the highest standard of worthiness, seeing the inevitable transformations that come with motherhood as something to be ashamed of. As a coach and wellness professional, I have come to understand how such a perspective can inadvertently contribute to body shaming. It appears that I advocated for embarrassment or correction of the remarkable journey of childbirth, instead of celebrating it.

This understanding brings forth a profound feeling of both regret and transparency. I feel compelled to rectify my previous statement. Childbirth is truly a remarkable experience—a profound reflection of the strength and beauty inherent in the female body. What could possibly motivate someone to overlook or dismiss the significant transformations that accompany the arrival of new life? It feels like I used to see these changes as a flaw instead of a source of pride.

As we navigate these emotional complexities, self-compassion becomes our greatest ally. It invites us to treat ourselves with the same kindness and understanding we would offer to a dear friend. By embracing this nurturing attitude we start to break down the barriers that hold us back from fully accepting our bodies just as beautiful they are right now. This acceptance not only nurtures our emotional well-being but also honors the incredible journey of motherhood and celebrates the resilient bodies that have carried us through this transformative experience.

Coming Full Circle: Understanding the Root of Body Idealization

As I dove deeper into my journey it became strikingly clear that my relentless pursuit of a pre-mom body wasn't just about achieving physical perfection—it was an attempt to mend deeper, unresolved wounds. I had convinced myself that sculpting my body into an ideal image was the path to feeling complete because, at a core level, I felt profoundly flawed. This sense of inadequacy extended beyond appearance, reflecting a loss of identity that started long before I became a mother.

I remember staring at myself in the mirror, fixating on every perceived flaw, pushing myself to sculpt perfectly defined arms and a chiseled abdomen. Each new milestone seemed to push the ideal further away, like a mirage just out of reach. I was chipping away at my body, hoping to reveal a masterpiece that always felt just beyond my grasp. But this obsession with physical perfection wasn't just about how I looked; it was a way to mask wounds that had never fully healed. Yes, another coping mechanism.

My struggle with fitness was a desperate attempt to regain control and self-worth, something that had been taken from me long ago. It became a façade—a defense mechanism against the overwhelming feelings of unworthiness and disconnection from my true self.

An old friend once observed that fitness was the only area in which I consistently followed through. She noticed that I struggled to maintain commitments in other areas of my life, like business ventures and personal projects. She wasn't criticizing my fitness journey, just saying it was the one thing I could control. And she was right. My focus on fitness was a reflection of the one thing I could reliably manage in a world where everything else felt chaotic. This obsession with fitness was my way of coping with unresolved traumas that made it difficult for me to follow through on other commitments, including our friendship. I wasn't trying to push her away; rather, my inability to connect and support others stemmed from my emotional struggles.

Realizing this has been a pivotal moment in my healing process. It has highlighted how deeply our struggles with body image are often tied to our deep emotional wounds. For many of us, the pursuit of an ideal appearance is not just about how we look; it's about seeking validation, healing old scars, and finding a lost sense of self.

Embracing self-compassion now means so much more than accepting my body as it is. It's about confronting and healing those deeper emotional scars and reconnecting with the authentic, evolving beauty of who I truly am inside. This journey has transformed my quest from an unattainable perfection to a celebration of my own unique story. To any mother who has felt this way, know that you are not alone. Your path to self-acceptance and healing is not just about the reflection in the mirror—it's about honoring the incredible person you are, both inside and out.

How childhood trauma can lead to increased inflammation later in life:

1. Stress Response System Activation:

- **Childhood trauma** activates the body's stress response system. When someone experiences trauma, their body releases stress hormones like **cortisol** and **adrenaline**.

- While these hormones are helpful in short bursts (like during an emergency), prolonged exposure due to ongoing stress or trauma can lead to dysregulation of the body's systems.

2. Inflammation Trigger:

- Chronic stress can trigger a persistent state of inflammation in the body. The stress response can cause the immune system to become overactive, leading to increased levels of inflammatory markers such as **C-reactive protein (CRP)** and **Interleukin-6 (IL-6)**.
- This inflammation is part of the body's way of responding to perceived threats, but when it's constant, it can start damaging tissues and organs.

3. Psychological Factors:

- Trauma can lead to mental health issues like **PTSD** and **depression**, which are also associated with higher inflammation levels. The emotional distress from these conditions can create a feedback loop that further raises inflammation.

4. Lifestyle Choices:

- Individuals with a history of trauma might engage in unhealthy coping mechanisms, such as poor diet, lack of exercise, or substance abuse. These lifestyle factors can also contribute to increased inflammation over time.

5. Biological Changes:

- Childhood trauma can affect how genes are expressed (a process called **epigenetics**), which may influence inflammation pathways. This means that the effects of trauma can be embedded in a person's biology, affecting their immune response even if the trauma occurred many years earlier.

6. Long-Term Health Consequences:

- Over time, chronic inflammation can lead to various health problems, including cardiovascular disease, autoimmune disorders, and other chronic conditions. It may also contribute to mental health issues, creating a cycle of distress.

Interactive Exercises

Exercise 1: Self-Compassion Journal

Purpose:
This exercise helps you connect with your inner thoughts and emotions, fostering a sense of safety and acceptance within you. By journaling, you'll create a safe space to explore your feelings without judgment.

Instructions:

1. **Set the Scene**

    Find a quiet, comfortable spot where you can write without distractions. Bring along your favorite journal or a notebook and perhaps a warm cup of tea. Allow yourself to settle in and take a few deep breaths.

2. **Reflective Prompt 1: Acknowledge Your Emotions**

    Write about a recent experience where you felt overwhelmed, stressed, or inadequate. Describe the situation in detail, focusing on how it made you feel both emotionally and physically.
    Example:

"The other day, I felt really stressed when I couldn't get everything done on my to-do list. My chest felt tight and I was short with the kids, which made me feel even worse…"

3. **Reflective Prompt 2: Reframe with Compassion**

   Now revisit the situation, but this time write as if you were comforting a close friend who was going through the same experience. What would you say to them? How would you help them see the situation from a kinder, more compassionate perspective?

   Example:

   "If I were talking to a friend, I'd remind her that she's doing her best and that it's okay to have days when everything doesn't go perfectly. I'd tell her that she's still a wonderful mom, even when things don't go as planned…"

4. **Reflective Prompt 3: Release the Guilt**

   Write about any guilt or self-criticism you've been holding on to. Imagine releasing it like a heavy weight you've been carrying. How does it feel to let go? What positive things can you say about yourself in this moment?

   Example:

   "I realize that I've been holding on to guilt about not being the 'perfect' mom. But I'm letting that go now because I know I'm doing my best. I'm learning, growing, and showing up for my kids, and that's what really matters…"

5. **Reflective Prompt 4: Set an Intention**

   End your journaling session by setting an intention for how you want to treat yourself moving forward. What's one small act of self-compassion you can commit to today?

   Example:

"Today, I'm going to give myself permission to rest when I need it. I'll remind myself that it's okay to take breaks and that my well-being is just as important as everything else on my to-do list."

Exercise 2: Self-Compassion Affirmations

Purpose:
This exercise helps reinforce positive self-talk and fosters a deeper connection to your sense of self-worth. By repeating affirmations you'll cultivate a habit of kindness toward yourself.

Instructions:

1. Create Your Affirmation Space
Find a calm, peaceful place where you can say your affirmations out loud. You might want to stand in front of a mirror, sit comfortably on the floor, or even take a walk outside.

2. Affirmation Creation
Below are some self-compassion affirmations to get you started. Feel free to modify them or create your own based on what resonates with you:

- "I am worthy of love and compassion."
- "I honor my emotions and give myself space to feel."
- "I am doing my best and that is enough."
- "I forgive myself for any mistakes I've made."
- "I am gentle with myself, just as I would be with a friend."
- "I embrace my imperfections as part of my unique journey."
- "I trust myself to make the best decisions for me and my family."
- "I deserve moments of peace and relaxation."
- "I am strong, capable, and resilient."

3. Daily Practice

Choose three affirmations that resonate with you most and repeat them every morning or before bed. Say each affirmation slowly, either out loud or silently, focusing on the meaning behind the words. Feel free to write them down and place them where you'll see them often, like on your mirror, fridge, or phone background.

4. Mindful Affirmation Practice

As you say each affirmation, take a deep breath in and out, allowing the words to sink in. Imagine the positive energy of each affirmation spreading throughout your body, filling you with a sense of calm and confidence.

5. Reflection

After a week of practicing your affirmations, take a few moments to reflect. How do you feel? Have these affirmations made a difference in your mood, mindset, or interactions with others? Write down any changes you've noticed in your journal or share them with a friend who's on a similar journey.

CHAPTER 14

The Weight of Your Own Story

You've probably heard it a million times: "Just let it go." But here's the truth they don't tell you—some things aren't easily let go of. Some things stick. They cling to the edges of your mind, shadowing every step you take, every decision you make. And for many of us, that thing, that sticky, unshakeable thing, is our childhood.

Grieving Your Childhood: A Necessary Step Toward Healing

Many mothers carry the weight of unresolved childhood trauma, often without realizing how deeply it affects their present lives. This grief isn't just about what happened to you, it's also about what didn't—the unconditional love, care, guidance, support, or safety you missed. Grieving your childhood is a crucial part of the healing process. It involves acknowledging the hurt and loss, allowing yourself to feel the pain, and giving yourself permission to mourn what was lost.

Grief is often misunderstood. It's not a linear process and it doesn't have a definitive endpoint. Instead, it's a journey that ebbs and flows. As you move through this grief you may experience a range of emotions—anger, sadness, confusion, relief. All of these feelings are valid and they are all part of the process of releasing the past to make space for healing and growth.

You might try to bury it under the busyness of motherhood, under the relentless to-do lists and constant demands, but there's always that moment—maybe it's in the quiet of the night when the house is finally still or maybe it's when you catch a glimpse of yourself in the mirror and realize you don't quite recognize the person staring back at you—there's that moment when it all comes flooding back. The childhood you never really got to grieve. The wounds that never truly healed.

You were supposed to be carefree. Innocent. You were supposed to feel safe and loved, to be nurtured into the person you were meant to become. But instead there was pain. Maybe it was a quiet kind of pain, creeping in through neglect, the absence of affection, or the burden of responsibilities too heavy for your small shoulders. Or maybe it was loud and violent, leaving marks on your skin and echoes in your mind.

Whatever it was, it shaped you. It influenced the way you see the world, the way you see yourself. It's there in the choices you make, the relationships you have, the way you mother your own children. It's the silent driver behind your fears and insecurities, behind that nagging voice that tells you you're not enough, that you'll never be enough.

But here's the thing—acknowledging this pain doesn't mean you're weak. It doesn't mean you're broken. It means you're human. And more importantly, it means you're ready to start healing. You see, the first step to reclaiming your life, to truly stepping into your power as a mother and as a woman, is to face the weight of your own story. To stop running from it. To stop pretending that it doesn't matter because it does. It always has.

The Loss of Identity in Motherhood: Finding Your True North

Motherhood is often heralded as a profound and transformative experience. Yet, what's less commonly discussed is the accompanying loss of identity that many mothers encounter. As you embrace the role of a mother, you might find that the person you once were—the woman with dreams, desires, and aspirations—feels like a distant memory or even lost altogether. This sense of loss can be disorienting and painful, but it doesn't signify the end of your identity. Instead, it's an invitation to gently rediscover and redefine who you really are.

Reconnecting with yourself requires more than just effort; it needs intention and compassion. It's about peeling away the layers of roles and responsibilities that have accumulated over time and finding your true north—the essence of you that exists beyond the role of motherhood. Finding your true north is about identifying and staying true to your core values, purpose, and guiding principles. It's a process of discovering what truly matters to you and aligning your life, decisions, and actions with that inner compass.

Here's what this thoughtful journey entails:

1. **Self-Discovery:** Gently exploring your strengths, passions, and what drives you. This involves introspection and reflection on your experiences and desires, helping you reconnect with the parts of you that may have been overshadowed by motherhood.

2. **Values Alignment:** Identifying and prioritizing your core values. These are the principles that guide your behavior and decisions. When your actions align with your values, you're more likely to feel fulfilled and authentic, nurturing a deeper sense of peace within you.

3. **Purpose:** Clarifying your life's purpose or mission. This broader sense of direction gives your life meaning beyond daily tasks and challenges, helping you navigate through the complexities of motherhood with a clear sense of what's truly important to you.

4. **Consistency:** Ensuring that your decisions and actions reflect your true north. This means making choices that are in harmony with your values and purpose, even when it's challenging. Consistency helps maintain a sense of integrity and direction, offering comfort and stability.

5. **Resilience:** Staying true to your true north can help you navigate difficulties and setbacks. It provides a sense of direction and stability, even in uncertain times, allowing you to move forward with a gentle strength.

Being intentional in this journey involves creating dedicated moments for reflection and growth. It means nurturing the aspects of you that might have been set aside. Set boundaries to protect time for self-discovery and prioritize your needs alongside those of your family. Engaging in mindfulness allows you to connect deeply with your thoughts, emotions, and desires, helping you rediscover your passions and the core of who you are.

This journey of intentional reconnection is a tender act of self-love and self-respect. It's about honoring your full humanity—not just as a mother but as a multifaceted individual with unique dreams, aspirations, and a distinct voice. By committing to this rediscovery, you're not only finding joy in being authentically yourself but also becoming the best version of you for those you love.

Reclaiming Your Identity: The Return to Dreams and Aspirations

Motherhood has a way of consuming you. It's easy to get so focused on being a good mother that you lose sight of your own needs, dreams, and story. Think of yourself as a teacup with an overflowing saucer. When your cup is brimming with self-care, joy, and fulfillment, it spills over into the saucer, allowing you to give generously without feeling drained.

Reclaiming your identity doesn't mean you love your children any less or that you're being selfish. In fact, it means quite the opposite. It's about acknowledging that you matter too and that your happiness, fulfillment, and sense of self are crucial components of being a good mother. By reclaiming your identity, you enrich your own life and give your children the best version of you—the one who is whole and alive.

So, who are you? Who were you before motherhood, before life happened to you? What are the parts of you that you've lost along the way? It's time to find them again. Remember what makes you feel alive, what brings you joy, what makes you uniquely you. When you reclaim your identity, you're not just doing it for yourself—you're doing it for your children too. You're showing them what it looks like to live fully, love fully, and be fully alive.

Consider the dreams and aspirations you once held. Maybe you wanted to travel the world, start a business, write a book, or simply have the freedom to pursue hobbies and passions. These dreams aren't gone; they're waiting for you to rediscover them. They are pieces of your identity that have been overshadowed by the demands of motherhood but are still an integral part of who you are.

Forgiveness: The Hardest Gift

Let's talk about forgiveness. Not the easy kind, the one that comes with an apology and a hug. No, let's dive into the kind of forgiveness that feels nearly impossible—the kind that asks you to let go of the anger, the hurt, and the betrayal that has been a part of your life for so long.

This kind of forgiveness isn't just about the other person. It's about you. It's about giving yourself the gift of freedom from the chains that bind you to your past. It's about making a decision that what happened to you will not dictate your future. It's about choosing peace over pain, love over hate.

You might wonder, *How do you forgive someone who never said they were sorry? How do you forgive when the wounds are still fresh and painful?* Start by acknowledging your pain. Let yourself feel the hurt, the anger, the sadness. Then, when you're ready, choose to let it go—not because they deserve it but because you do. Forgiveness is not a one-time act; it's an ongoing process of letting go of pain and anger, step by step.

I understand this deeply because I experienced it myself. When I traveled to Manila to reconnect with my father—a man I hadn't seen in 24 years—I embarked on more than just a physical journey. It was an emotional pilgrimage to confront years of unresolved pain. When we finally met, I made a choice that was both monumental and freeing: I forgave him. It wasn't just about the act itself; it felt like lifting a thousand-pound weight off my shoulders. For years, I had carried heavy stones in a metaphorical backpack, each one symbolizing a piece of my unresolved grief. That day, those stones were finally put down. I was no longer shackled by a story that had defined me for so long.

That moment didn't just close a chapter; it opened a new one. It set me on a path where dreams that once felt out of reach became attainable. The projects I'm working on now, including this book, are a direct result of that liberating experience. They stand as a testament to the power of forgiveness and the possibility of new beginnings. What once seemed like distant dreams are now vibrant realities, showing that, no matter how heavy your burdens may seem, there is always hope.

For mothers, embracing forgiveness can be transformative—not just for your own life but for the lives of your children. Forgiving is one of the greatest gifts you can give yourself. It creates a more loving, understanding environment for your family. Remember, forgiveness is a journey, not a destination. It takes time and commitment and it's something you choose every day. With each act of forgiveness, you reclaim a little bit of your power, a little bit of your life.

You'll find that the weight of your past isn't as heavy as it once was. You'll find that you can breathe a little easier, love a little more freely, and live more fully.

By letting go of past hurts you open the door to a future where you can nurture yourself and your children, creating a legacy of strength and resilience.

Faith and Divine Guidance: The Strength Beyond You

If you only read one chapter in this book, let it be this one. You are not your past. You are not your pain. You are not the sum of what happened to you. You are so much more than that. You are a mother, yes, but you are also a person—a person with a story that deserves to be heard, a person with dreams that deserve to be realized, a person with a life that deserves to be lived.

The strength you possess, the resilience that carries you through even the toughest of times, is not solely the result of your own efforts or abilities. It is the gentle grace of a higher power that has been guiding you, supporting you, and holding you close. For me, this source of strength is my faith in God. Jeremiah 1:5 (NIV) offers a comforting reminder: "Before I formed you in the womb I knew you, before you were born I set you apart; I appointed you as a prophet to the nations." This verse speaks to a profound truth: God meticulously crafted your life even before you took your first breath, knowing you in ways you might not yet fully understand.

Yes, we have all faced sorrowful and painful moments, times when the weight of our struggles felt almost too much to bear. Yet, even in these trials, we are reminded that every experience, every challenge, and every triumph is part of His greater plan. This plan, designed with love, supports our growth and draws us closer to our true potential. You are cherished beyond measure and each step of your journey is guided by a purpose that is deeply personal and profoundly significant.

In the moments when the weight of your story feels overwhelming, remember this: Everything that has happened and everything that will happen is because He knows us intimately and desires the best for us. His wisdom is infinite, and His love is unwavering. Trust that He is guiding you through this journey, leading you toward healing and wholeness. Embrace the belief that He has not made a mistake in your life's path and that every step, even the painful ones, is drawing you closer to the person He intended you to be.

So, take the first step. Acknowledge the weight of your story and then start to let it go. Start to reclaim the parts of you that you've lost, start to forgive the people who have hurt you, and start to live the life you deserve. Above all, forgive yourself.

You deserve to be happy. You deserve to be whole. You deserve to be free. And, most importantly, you deserve to be you. With faith as your guide, you have the strength to heal, to grow, and to embrace the beautiful future that awaits you.

BONUS CHAPTER

Tools for Healing: Practical Techniques for Transformation

Healing from trauma, especially one from your childhood, is a deeply personal journey and finding the right tools can make all the difference. In this chapter, I share a collection of techniques and practices that have been instrumental in my own healing process. Each of these tools has helped me address emotional wounds, manage stress, and cultivate a healthier, more balanced life. And, truthfully, they have led me here in writing this book for you. My hope is that by sharing these methods you'll find valuable resources that resonate with your own journey.

NLP Techniques

- **Anchoring**: Think about a time when you felt really calm and happy, maybe while enjoying a cup of tea or listening to your favorite song. You can create an anchor by squeezing a stress ball or placing your hand over your heart while you're in that peaceful moment. Later, when you're feeling overwhelmed, use that same gesture to bring back those calming feelings. It's like having your own little reset button!

- **Swish Pattern**: This technique is great for shifting your mindset. If you find yourself worrying about a challenging situation, visualize that worry as a dark cloud. Then quickly replace that image with something bright and positive, like a sunny day or a happy family moment. The more you practice this the easier it gets to let go of those worries and embrace the good!

- **Reframing**: Whenever you're faced with a difficult situation—maybe a tough day with the kids or a parenting mistake—try to reframe it. Instead of saying, "I can't believe I messed up," think, *This is a chance to learn and grow.* Shifting your perspective can help you see challenges as opportunities rather than setbacks.
- **Meta Model**: This technique encourages you to question any negative beliefs you might have about yourself. If you catch yourself saying, "I'm not a good mom," ask yourself, "What makes me feel that way?" or "What evidence do I have to support that?" You might be surprised to find that you're doing a lot better than you think!
- **Future Pacing**: Imagine a situation you're anxious about, like a family gathering or a school event. Picture yourself handling it with confidence and grace. Visualize everything going smoothly, from the conversations to the fun moments. This technique helps you prepare mentally, making it easier to approach those situations with a positive mindset.

Deep Breathing

Deep breathing exercises are a simple yet powerful way to manage stress and promote relaxation. By focusing on your breath you activate the parasympathetic nervous system, which helps counteract the effects of stress.

Diaphragmatic Breathing: Breathe in deeply through your nose, allowing your abdomen to rise. Exhale slowly through your mouth, feeling your abdomen fall. Repeat for a few minutes to calm your mind and body.

Box Breathing: Inhale for four seconds, hold for four seconds, exhale for four seconds, and hold again for four seconds. This technique can help regulate your breathing and reduce anxiety.

Tapping (Emotional Freedom Techniques)

Tapping, or Emotional Freedom Techniques (EFT), combines cognitive therapy with acupressure. By tapping on specific points on the body while focusing on a negative emotion or thought you can help release emotional blocks.

Basic Tapping Procedure: Identify the issue, tap on the specific acupressure points (such as the side of the hand, top of the head, and under the eyes), and repeat a phrase that acknowledges the problem and affirms self-acceptance.

The Butterfly Hug

The Butterfly Hug is a simple self-soothing technique that helps manage emotions, reduce anxiety, and promote relaxation. It's great for both children and adults and can be practiced anywhere.

How to Practice the Butterfly Hug:

1. **Find a Comfortable Space**: Choose a quiet, safe area to relax.

2. **Cross Your Arms**: Bring your arms across your chest, resting your hands on your shoulders.

3. **Begin Tapping**: Gently tap your shoulders alternately, mimicking the flapping of butterfly wings. Choose a rhythm that feels comfortable.

4. **Focus on Your Breathing**: Inhale deeply through your nose, hold for a moment, and exhale through your mouth to enhance the calming effect.

5. **Set an Intention**: Think about what you're feeling or set a positive intention.

6. **Continue for a Few Minutes**: Practice for as long as feels right—typically a couple of minutes or longer.

How and Why the Butterfly Hug Works:

- **Bilateral Stimulation**: The alternating tapping engages both sides of the body, which can calm the brain and reduce anxiety.
- **Nervous System Activation**: Tapping activates the parasympathetic nervous system, promoting relaxation and reducing heart rate and blood pressure.
- **Mindfulness**: Focusing on your breath and the tapping brings you into the present moment, quieting racing thoughts.
- **Emotional Regulation**: Over time, this practice helps reinforce your ability to manage overwhelming emotions.

Binaural Beats

Binaural beats are a fascinating auditory illusion that happens when you listen to two slightly different frequencies in each ear. For example, if one ear hears a sound at 200 Hz and the other hears a sound at 210 Hz, your brain creates the perception of a third sound at 10 Hz (the difference between the two). This clever trick can help synchronize brainwave activity, promoting relaxation, focus, or even better sleep.

How and Why Binaural Beats Work:

- **Brainwave Synchronization**: When you listen to binaural beats, your brain tries to make sense of the two different frequencies. This process encourages your brain to align its electrical activity (or brainwaves)

with the perceived beat. This means you can influence your mental state in a really positive way!
- **Auditory Processing**: Your auditory system picks up on these beats, which can impact your emotions and how you think. By listening to binaural beats you can tap into specific brainwave states that help you relax, focus, or feel more creative.
- **Neurotransmitter Release**: Binaural beats might also help your brain release feel-good chemicals like serotonin and dopamine. These neurotransmitters play key roles in lifting your mood and promoting relaxation.

Brainwave Frequencies and Their Effects:

- **Delta Waves (1–4 Hz)**: These low-frequency waves are all about promoting deep sleep and relaxation. If you're looking for a restful night, these are your go-to beats!
- **Theta Waves (4–8 Hz)**: Associated with deep meditation and bursts of creativity, theta waves can enhance your intuition and emotional connection. They create a wonderful space for relaxation and insight.
- **Alpha Waves (8–14 Hz)**: These moderate frequencies help you unwind and reduce stress. They're perfect for achieving a calm and alert state, often experienced during light meditation.

Meditation

Meditation is a powerful practice that helps you center your mind and cultivate a sense of peace. It's not just about sitting in silence; it's about training your brain to focus and gain a deeper understanding of your thoughts and feelings. Whether you're just starting out or you've been meditating for a while, it can be a wonderful way to improve your overall well-being.

How and Why Meditation Works

- **Focus and Clarity**: During meditation, you focus on your breath, a mantra, or even a specific thought. This concentration helps quiet the mind, leading to a relaxed state. Scientific studies have shown that mindfulness meditation can significantly lower stress levels and reduce anxiety by decreasing cortisol, the stress hormone.
- **Mindfulness and Emotional Awareness**: Many meditation practices promote mindfulness, encouraging you to be fully present in the moment. This awareness allows you to observe your thoughts and feelings without judgment, which can boost emotional resilience. Research indicates that practicing mindfulness can help improve emotional regulation and lift your mood.
- **Physiological Benefits**: Meditation can also bring about positive changes in your body. Studies show that mindfulness meditation can lower blood pressure and improve heart rate variability, both signs of better heart health. These changes help foster a state of relaxation and contribute to overall wellness.

What Happens in the Brain During Meditation

When you meditate, several fascinating changes occur in your brain that enhance both your mental and emotional health:

1. **Increased Gray Matter**: Regular meditation is linked to an increase in gray matter density in areas of the brain responsible for memory, emotional regulation, and self-awareness. This means that, over time, meditation can physically change your brain to better handle emotions and thoughts.

2. **Reduced Activity in the Default Mode Network (DMN)**: The DMN is active when your mind wanders or ruminates on the past and future. During meditation, activity in this network decreases,

allowing you to focus more on the present moment. This shift can lead to a reduction in anxiety and stress.

3. **Enhanced Connectivity**: Meditation enhances the connections between different brain regions, improving communication among them. This can lead to better emotional regulation and cognitive flexibility, helping you respond to situations more effectively.

4. **Increased Activity in the Prefrontal Cortex**: This area of the brain is responsible for executive functions like decision-making, attention, and self-control. Meditation boosts activity in this region, enabling you to manage stress and improve focus more effectively.

5. **Emotional Regulation**: Changes in brain activity during meditation help regulate emotions. Research shows that meditation strengthens the connection between the amygdala (the brain's emotion center) and the prefrontal cortex, allowing for better emotional responses and reducing impulsivity.

Benefits of Meditation

- **Reduces Stress and Anxiety**: Regular meditation practice can help you manage stress and anxiety effectively. By focusing on the present you create distance from worries, allowing for a calmer mindset.
- **Enhances Emotional Well-Being**: Research shows that meditation can improve your mood and increase feelings of happiness. It can also help alleviate symptoms of depression, leading to a more positive outlook on life.
- **Improves Concentration and Focus**: Meditation helps sharpen your attention and enhances your ability to concentrate. Studies suggest that mindfulness practices can boost your focus and cognitive flexibility, making it easier to tackle daily tasks.

- **Promotes Better Sleep**: If you struggle with sleep, meditation might be your solution. Studies indicate that mindfulness meditation significantly improves sleep quality, especially for those who experience insomnia or sleep disturbances.

Getting Started with Meditation

1. **Choose a Quiet Space**: Find a comfortable spot where you won't be interrupted.

2. **Set a Time Limit**: If you're new, start with just 5–10 minutes. You can gradually increase the time as you get more comfortable.

3. **Focus on Your Breath**: Close your eyes and take a few deep breaths. Pay attention to how your breath feels as it flows in and out.

4. **Gently Redirect Your Thoughts**: If your mind starts to wander, gently bring your focus back to your breath or your chosen point of focus. It's completely normal for thoughts to come up!

5. **Practice Regularly**: Try to make meditation a daily habit, even if it's just for a few minutes. Consistency is key to experiencing the benefits.

Journaling

Journaling is a wonderful practice that can be a real game-changer for your emotional well-being. It's more than just putting pen to paper; it's a chance for you to dive deep into your thoughts and feelings, helping you process what's going on in your life. Whether you're looking to understand yourself better or simply need an outlet for your emotions, journaling can be a safe space for self-reflection and growth.

How and Why Journaling Works

- **Reflective Journaling**: This is all about writing down your daily experiences and how they made you feel. By reflecting on your thoughts and emotions, you can start to recognize patterns and triggers in your life. This practice not only helps clarify your feelings but can also reveal insights about what brings you joy or stress. Research shows that expressive writing can significantly reduce anxiety and improve mood, making it a valuable tool for emotional regulation.
- **Gratitude Journaling**: This involves taking a few moments each day to list things you're grateful for. Focusing on gratitude shifts your attention away from negativity and helps you appreciate the positive aspects of life. Studies have found that practicing gratitude can enhance overall happiness and satisfaction while reducing symptoms of depression. It's a beautiful way to foster a more positive mindset and remind yourself of the good things, even on tough days.

Getting Started with Journaling

1. **Choose Your Medium**: Decide whether you prefer writing in a traditional notebook or typing on your computer. The important thing is to find a method that feels comfortable for you.

2. **Set Aside Time**: Try to carve out a few minutes each day, whether it's in the morning with your coffee or before bed to unwind. Consistency can help make journaling a fulfilling habit.

3. **Be Honest and Open**: Don't worry about grammar or style. Write freely about your thoughts and feelings. This is your space to express yourself without judgment.

4. **Experiment with Different Styles**: You might find that some days you prefer reflective journaling while other days gratitude journaling feels right. There's no wrong way to do it!

5. **Review Your Entries**: Occasionally, look back at your previous entries. This reflection can reveal how far you've come and offer valuable insights into your emotional journey.

Foam Rolling

Foam rolling is a fantastic self-care technique that can help release tension in your muscles and improve overall body function. Think of it as a personal massage you can do anytime, anywhere! By rolling a foam roller over different areas of your body you're working out those tight spots and knots, which can lead to reduced soreness and increased flexibility.

How It Works: When you use a foam roller, you're applying pressure to your muscles, which helps increase blood flow and release built-up tension. This process, known as self-myofascial release, can alleviate pain and improve your range of motion. Plus, taking time to care for your body like this can feel incredibly nurturing and restorative.

Epsom Salt Baths

Epsom salt baths are a simple yet effective way to unwind and soothe both your body and mind. Epsom salt, which is actually magnesium sulfate, can be absorbed through your skin, helping to relax muscles and reduce inflammation.

How It Works: When you soak in a warm bath with Epsom salt, the magnesium can help lower cortisol levels, which is the stress hormone. This leads to feelings of relaxation and tranquility. Adding calming scents like lavender can enhance the experience, creating a spa-like atmosphere at home.

Taking time for yourself in a warm bath is not just about relaxation; it's a lovely way to practice self-care and let go of the day's stress.

Dancing

Even if you have two left feet, it is such a joyful and uplifting way to express yourself and connect with your emotions. It's not just about the fun of moving to music; it's also a therapeutic activity that can boost your mood and relieve stress.

- **Freestyle Dance**: Put on your favorite tunes and let yourself move freely! Don't worry about how it looks; just enjoy the sensation of moving your body to the rhythm. This kind of dance encourages you to focus on the joy of movement, allowing you to express your emotions physically and shake off any negativity.
- **Dance Therapy**: If you want to explore dance in a more structured way, consider joining a dance therapy group. Here, you can use movement as a form of emotional healing and self-expression. Dance therapy often combines creative movement with therapeutic techniques, helping you process emotions and connect with others in a supportive environment.

Why It Works: Dancing releases endorphins, those feel-good hormones that can instantly lift your spirits. Plus, the physical activity helps reduce tension and anxiety, making it another powerful tool for your emotional well-being.

Jumping

Jumping can be a transformative practice for those healing from trauma, offering a powerful outlet for releasing pent-up emotions. It's more than just physical movement; it's a way to reconnect with joy and reclaim your sense of freedom. Whether you're seeking a burst of energy or a means to shake off lingering stress, jumping can serve as a vital tool for emotional healing.

How and Why Jumping Works

Release of Endorphins: When you jump, your body releases endorphins, the "feel-good" hormones that can significantly elevate your mood and counteract feelings of stress and anxiety. For someone healing from trauma, this natural high can create a sense of empowerment and vitality, helping to counteract feelings of despair.

Physical Expression: Jumping allows for the physical expression of emotions that may be difficult to articulate. It provides an opportunity to let go of tension and embrace a sense of freedom, fostering a positive mindset as you navigate your healing journey.

Boosts Energy Levels: The act of jumping increases blood flow and oxygen levels, leading to enhanced energy and alertness. This boost can help you confront daily challenges with renewed strength, promoting resilience in your healing process.

Rocking

Rocking is a soothing practice that can bring comfort and stability to those recovering from trauma. Whether you find solace in rocking in a chair or swaying gently, this rhythmic motion fosters relaxation and helps ground you in the present moment. It's a gentle way to create a safe space for self-reflection and healing.

How and Why Rocking Works

Promotes Calmness: The rhythmic motion of rocking can activate the body's relaxation response, lowering heart rate and alleviating stress. For trauma survivors, this calming effect can be especially beneficial, helping to ease feelings of anxiety and create a sense of safety.

Sensory Regulation: Rocking engages your body in a way that helps regulate sensory input, which can be particularly helpful for those who feel overwhelmed by their surroundings. This gentle motion provides a means to manage emotions and find balance amidst chaos.

Emotional Comfort: The act of rocking often evokes feelings of safety and nurturing, reminiscent of childhood comforts. This emotional connection can enhance overall well-being, offering a refuge where you can explore and process your feelings during your healing journey.

"VOO" Sound

Making the "VOO" sound introduces a vocal element that can significantly aid in trauma healing. This simple sound creates vibrations that resonate within, promoting a deeper connection between your body and mind while also engaging the vagus nerve, a key player in regulating your body's stress response.

How and Why the "VOO" Sound Works

Vocal Expression: The "VOO" sound releases energy and connects you with difficult emotions. This vocalization can soothe you, focusing your mind on the sound and vibration for calm.

Vagus Nerve Engagement: The vagus nerve, essential for relaxation, is stimulated by the "VOO" sound, promoting safety and reducing anxiety. Activating it can lower heart rate and cortisol levels, aiding healing.

Mind-Body Connection: This practice enhances mindfulness, increasing awareness of your emotions and sensations. Tuning into the "VOO" vibrations improves emotional regulation, empowering your healing journey and helping you navigate trauma with clarity and resilience.

How to "VOO"

1. **Find a Comfortable Space:** Choose a quiet place where you feel safe and relaxed, free from distractions.

2. **Relax Your Body:** Take a few deep breaths to help release any tension in your body. You might want to sit or lie down in a comfortable position.

3. **Inhale Deeply:** Take a deep breath in through your nose, filling your lungs completely.

4. **Vocalize the "VOO" Sound:** As you exhale, let out a gentle "VOO" sound, feeling the vibrations in your chest and throat. You can vary the pitch and intensity, experimenting with what feels best for you.

5. **Focus on the Sensation:** Pay attention to how the sound resonates within your body. Notice any shifts in your emotional state or physical sensations as you continue to vocalize the sound.

6. **Repeat as Needed:** You can repeat the "VOO" sound for several minutes, allowing yourself to become immersed in this experience. If you feel your mind wandering, gently bring your focus back to the sound and vibrations.

7. **Reflect:** When you finish, take a moment to reflect on how you feel. Notice changes in your mood or physical state and give yourself permission to process those feelings.

Weight Lifting and Other Fitness Formats

Weight Lifting

Weight lifting strengthens both body and mind, building resilience, boosting self-esteem, and managing stress. It enhances muscle strength, metabolism, and endorphin levels, improving mood and well-being. Start with light weights, focus on form, and gradually increase the weight as you gain strength.

Other Formats

Incorporating various fitness formats can further enhance physical and mental health:

- **Yoga**: Promotes flexibility, mindfulness, and relaxation. It can help reduce stress and improve mental clarity.
- **Pilates**: Focuses on core strength, flexibility, and body awareness. It can improve posture and relieve tension in the body.
- **CrossFit**: A high-intensity workout combining weightlifting, cardio, and functional movements. It builds strength and endurance while fostering a sense of community.
- **Barre**: A fusion of ballet, Pilates, and yoga that emphasizes small, controlled movements. It helps tone muscles and improve flexibility.
- **Rowing**: A full-body workout that enhances cardiovascular fitness and strengthens muscles. It can be both an individual and a team activity.
- **Cycling**: Offers a low-impact way to build cardiovascular endurance and leg strength. It can be done indoors or outdoors, providing flexibility in your workout routine.

Each of these formats provides unique benefits that contribute to overall health and wellness. By exploring different types of exercise you can find what resonates with you best. Just remember to enjoy these activities and participating in them should never feel like a chore!

Progressive Muscle Relaxation

Progressive Muscle Relaxation (PMR) is a technique that involves tensing and then relaxing each muscle group in your body. This practice can help you become more aware of physical tension and promote overall relaxation.

How It Works: By intentionally tensing and releasing muscles, you create a contrast that helps you recognize and let go of tension in your body. This technique encourages relaxation and can reduce feelings of stress and anxiety.

Getting Started with PMR:

1. **Find a Quiet Space**: Sit or lie down in a comfortable position.

2. **Start from the Feet**: Begin by tensing the muscles in your feet for a few seconds. Notice the tension.

3. **Release**: Let go of the tension and feel the relaxation.

4. **Move Up the Body**: Gradually move to other muscle groups (calves, thighs, abdomen, arms, shoulders, and face), tensing and relaxing each one.

5. **Breathe**: Take deep breaths as you do this to enhance the feeling of relaxation.

Sleep Optimization
(Detailed how to and tips in Chapter 6.)

Quality sleep is essential for healing and overall health. Poor sleep can exacerbate stress and emotional difficulties.

Sleep Hygiene: Establish a regular sleep schedule, create a restful environment, and avoid screens before bedtime.

Art Therapy

A creative approach that allows you to express your emotions through various art forms—whether it's painting, drawing, pottery, or crafting. It provides a non-verbal outlet for feelings and can promote healing and self-discovery.

How It Works: Engaging in creative expression activates different parts of the brain, encouraging emotional release and helping you process experiences. Art therapy can help reduce anxiety and improve emotional well-being.

Getting Started with Art Therapy:

1. **Gather Your Supplies**: You don't need anything fancy! Just grab some paper, crayons, markers, or paints.

2. **Set Your Intention**: Decide if you want to express a specific emotion or simply create for the joy of it.

3. **Allow Free Expression**: Don't worry about the outcome. Just let your emotions guide your creativity. Draw, paint, or create whatever comes to mind.

4. **Reflect**: After you've created something, take a moment to reflect on how it made you feel. You might want to write about your experience or simply enjoy the piece you've created.

Nature Walks

How many times have you gone on a walk and instantly felt better? Spending time in nature has been shown to reduce stress, boost mood, and enhance overall well-being. Being in nature can lower cortisol levels (the stress hormone), enhance mood, and improve focus. The sights, sounds, and smells of nature engage your senses and help you feel more grounded and connected.

Find a nearby park or trail and walk mindfully, observing your surroundings and breathing deeply to relax. Afterward, take a moment to reflect on how you feel, maybe jotting down your thoughts in a journal.

Supplements for Emotional Healing

In the journey toward emotional healing, various supplements can play a supportive role in enhancing mental well-being. While this section highlights several supplements that have personally benefited me and others I have worked with, it's essential to remember that this list is not exhaustive. Each individual's body responds differently and what works for one person may not work for another. Always consult with a healthcare professional before introducing any new supplements into your routine to ensure they align with your specific needs and health conditions. By combining these supplements with a balanced diet, mindfulness practices, and professional guidance you can create a more holistic approach to emotional healing.

1. Antioxidants and Anti-Inflammatories

Antioxidants help combat oxidative stress, which can impact mental and emotional health. Here are several key antioxidants that may support emotional healing:

- **Grapeseed Extract**
    - **Benefits**: Improves circulation, enhances cognitive function, supports skin health.
    - **How It Works**: Rich in proanthocyanidins, it neutralizes free radicals and reduces inflammation.

- **Curcumin (from Turmeric)**
    - **Benefits**: Reduces inflammation, may improve mood, and supports cognitive function.

- o **How It Works**: Acts as a potent antioxidant and anti-inflammatory agent, inhibiting pro-inflammatory cytokines and enhancing brain-derived neurotrophic factor (BDNF) levels.

- **Green Tea Extract (EGCG)**
  - o **Benefits**: Supports cognitive function, reduces stress, and may improve mood.
  - o **How It Works**: Contains epigallocatechin gallate (EGCG), which protects neurons from oxidative stress and promotes brain health.

- **Vitamin C**
  - o **Benefits**: Supports immune function, reduces fatigue, and may improve mood.
  - o **How It Works**: A powerful antioxidant that helps reduce oxidative stress and is essential for neurotransmitter synthesis, including serotonin.

- **Vitamin E**
  - o **Benefits**: Protects cells from oxidative damage, supports skin health.
  - o **How It Works**: Acts as a fat-soluble antioxidant, protecting cell membranes from oxidative stress, which can positively influence mood and overall health.

- **Alpha-Lipoic Acid (ALA)**
  - o **Benefits**: Supports metabolic health and may improve symptoms of anxiety and depression.
  - o **How It Works**: Functions as both a fat-soluble and water-soluble antioxidant, regenerating other antioxidants like vitamins C and E, and reducing oxidative stress.

- **Coenzyme Q10 (CoQ10)**
  - **Benefits**: Supports energy production and may improve mood.
  - **How It Works**: Acts as an antioxidant in the mitochondria, enhancing cellular energy production and reducing oxidative damage.

- **Astaxanthin**
  - **Benefits**: Protects brain health and supports emotional well-being.
  - **How It Works**: A carotenoid with potent antioxidant properties that can cross the blood-brain barrier, reducing neuroinflammation and oxidative stress.

- **Resveratrol**
  - **Benefits**: Supports heart health, may improve mood, and has anti-inflammatory effects.
  - **How It Works**: Found in grapes and berries, it reduces oxidative stress and inflammation in the brain, potentially improving cognitive function and emotional resilience.

- **Selenium**
  - **Benefits**: Supports mood and cognitive function, may improve overall well-being.
  - **How It Works**: Acts as an antioxidant, protecting cells from oxidative damage, and plays a crucial role in thyroid function, which can influence mood.

- **Quercetin**
  - **Benefits**: Reduces inflammation and may support emotional health.

- o **How It Works**: A flavonoid that combats oxidative stress and promotes overall health by reducing inflammation and supporting immune function.

- **Bilberry Extract**
  - o **Benefits**: Supports eye health and may enhance cognitive function.
  - o **How It Works**: Rich in anthocyanins, which possess strong antioxidant properties, potentially protecting brain cells from oxidative damage.

- **Milk Thistle (Silymarin)**
  - o **Benefits**: Supports liver health, may improve mood, and provides antioxidant protection.
  - o **How It Works**: Contains silymarin, which protects liver cells from oxidative stress and enhances detoxification, benefiting overall emotional well-being.

2. Adaptogens

- **Ashwagandha**
  - o **Benefits**: Reduces stress and anxiety, enhances energy levels, improves mood.
  - o **How It Works**: Modulates cortisol levels, promoting a balanced stress response.

- **Rhodiola Rosea**
  - o **Benefits**: Improves mental performance, reduces fatigue, enhances resilience to stress.
  - o **How It Works**: Regulates neurotransmitters and enhances cellular energy production.

- **Holy Basil (Tulsi)**
  - **Benefits**: Reduces stress, improves mood, enhances mental clarity.
  - **How It Works**: Modulates stress hormones and promotes a sense of well-being.

3. **Amino Acids**

- **L-Arginine**
  - **Benefits**: Enhances blood flow, may improve exercise performance.
  - **How It Works**: Converts to nitric oxide, which dilates blood vessels.

- **L-Citrulline**
  - **Benefits**: Reduces muscle soreness, improves exercise endurance.
  - **How It Works**: Boosts nitric oxide levels.

- **L-Lysine**
  - **Benefits**: Supports immune function, reduces anxiety.
  - **How It Works**: Essential for protein synthesis and neurotransmitter function.

- **L-Carnitine**
  - **Benefits**: Supports fat metabolism, enhances energy levels.
  - **How It Works**: Transports fatty acids into mitochondria for energy production.

- **Taurine**
  - **Benefits**: Supports mood and cognitive function, may reduce anxiety.

- **How It Works**: Regulates neurotransmitters and promotes a calming effect.

4. Other Key Supplements

- **N-Acetyl Cysteine (NAC)**
  - **Benefits**: Supports emotional regulation, reduces anxiety symptoms.
  - **How It Works**: Boosts glutathione levels, a powerful antioxidant.

- **Beta-Alanine**
  - **Benefits**: Enhances exercise performance, reduces fatigue.
  - **How It Works**: Increases carnosine levels in muscles, buffering acid.

- **GABA (Gamma-Aminobutyric Acid)**
  - **Benefits**: Promotes relaxation, reduces feelings of overwhelm.
  - **How It Works**: Acts as an inhibitory neurotransmitter, calming the nervous system.

- **Magnesium**
  - **Benefits**: Reduces anxiety, supports sleep, improves mood.
  - **How It Works**: Regulates neurotransmitters and promotes relaxation.

- **Omega-3 Fatty Acids (EPA, DHA)**
  - **Benefits**: Supports brain health, reduces anxiety and depression.
  - **How It Works**: Increases levels of serotonin and dopamine, contributing to improved mood.

5. Herbal Supplements

- **Chamomile**
  - **Benefits**: Promotes relaxation and aids sleep.
  - **How It Works**: Has mild sedative properties that help reduce anxiety.

- **Passionflower**
  - **Benefits**: Reduces anxiety and improves sleep quality.
  - **How It Works**: Increases GABA levels, promoting relaxation.

- **St. John's Wort**
  - **Benefits**: May alleviate mild depression and anxiety.
  - **How It Works**: Affects serotonin levels and other neurotransmitters.

- **Evening Primrose Powder**
  - **Benefits**: May help with mood swings and emotional balance.
  - **How It Works**: Contains gamma-linolenic acid (GLA), which supports hormone balance and reduces inflammation.

6. Mushroom Extracts

- **Organic Reishi Mushroom**
  - **Benefits**: Reduces stress, supports sleep, enhances overall well-being.
  - **How It Works**: Contains adaptogenic properties that help regulate cortisol levels and promote relaxation.

- **Organic Cordyceps Mushroom**
  - **Benefits**: Increases energy and stamina, may improve mood.
  - **How It Works**: Enhances oxygen utilization and promotes blood flow.

- **Organic Shiitake Mushroom**
    - **Benefits**: Supports immune function and overall health.
    - **How It Works**: Contains polysaccharides that promote immune health and may improve mood.

- **Organic Lion's Mane Mushroom**
    - **Benefits**: Supports cognitive function, may reduce anxiety and depression.
    - **How It Works**: Promotes nerve growth factor (NGF) production, which supports brain health.

- **Green Coffee Bean Extract**
    - **Benefits**: May improve mood and cognitive function.
    - **How It Works**: Contains chlorogenic acid, which can help regulate blood sugar levels and has antioxidant properties.

- **Morinda Citrifolia (Noni)**
    - **Benefits**: Supports immune function and overall wellness.
    - **How It Works**: Contains antioxidants and compounds that may improve mood and reduce inflammation.

7. Vitamins and Minerals

A comprehensive list of vitamins and minerals that support emotional and mental health:

- **Vitamin D**
    - **Benefits**: Supports mood regulation and overall mental health.
    - **How It Works**: Influences serotonin levels and brain function.

- **Vitamin B Complex**
    - **Benefits**: Supports energy levels, brain health, and emotional balance.

- o **How It Works**: Essential for neurotransmitter synthesis and metabolism.

- **Folate (Vitamin B9)**
  - o **Benefits**: Supports mental health and emotional stability.
  - o **How It Works**: Crucial for DNA synthesis and neurotransmitter production.

- **Vitamin B12**
  - o **Benefits**: Supports nerve health and may improve mood.
  - o **How It Works**: Essential for red blood cell formation and neurological function.

- **Vitamin B6**
  - o **Benefits**: Aids in neurotransmitter production and may alleviate depression.
  - o **How It Works**: Converts tryptophan to serotonin, influencing mood.

- **Selenium**
  - o **Benefits**: Supports mood and cognitive function, may improve overall well-being.
  - o **How It Works**: Acts as an antioxidant, protecting cells from oxidative damage.

- **Zinc**
  - o **Benefits**: Supports immune function and may improve mood.
  - o **How It Works**: Involved in neurotransmitter function and can influence serotonin levels.

- **Iron**
  - o **Benefits**: Supports energy levels and cognitive function.

- o **How It Works**: Essential for oxygen transport and metabolism, influencing overall energy and mood.

- **Calcium**
  - o **Benefits**: Supports nerve transmission and may improve mood.
  - o **How It Works**: Plays a crucial role in neurotransmitter release and brain function.

- **Potassium**
  - o **Benefits**: Helps maintain nerve function and muscle contractions.
  - o **How It Works**: Regulates fluid balance and supports cellular function, impacting mood stability.

- **Magnesium**
  - o **Benefits**: Reduces anxiety, supports sleep, and improves mood.
  - o **How It Works**: Regulates neurotransmitters and promotes relaxation.

Biohacking with Food

List of Anti-Inflammatory and Nutrient-Dense Foods for Healing

1. Fruits

- **Berries** (e.g., blueberries, strawberries, raspberries): High in antioxidants and vitamin C, which help combat oxidative stress and inflammation. Antioxidants may also support brain health, which is essential for processing emotions and healing from trauma.
- **Cherries**: Contain anthocyanins that have anti-inflammatory effects, potentially reducing anxiety and enhancing mood.

- **Pineapple**: Contains bromelain, an enzyme that may help reduce inflammation and support digestive health, contributing to overall well-being.
- **Oranges**: Rich in vitamin C, which can help lower cortisol levels and combat stress.
- **Apples**: High in fiber and quercetin, an antioxidant that can help stabilize mood and reduce anxiety.
- **Grapes**: Contain resveratrol, which has been linked to reduced inflammation and improved brain function.

2. Vegetables

- **Leafy Greens** (e.g., spinach, kale, Swiss chard): Packed with vitamins, minerals, and antioxidants that combat oxidative stress and may enhance mental clarity, crucial for emotional healing.
- **Broccoli**: Contains sulforaphane, which has neuroprotective effects and may help mitigate anxiety.
- **Beets**: Rich in betalains, which have anti-inflammatory properties and support healthy circulation and mood regulation.
- **Bell Peppers**: High in vitamin C and antioxidants, which can aid in reducing stress levels and improving overall mood.
- **Carrots**: Rich in beta-carotene, which has been associated with improved mood and cognitive function.
- **Cauliflower**: Contains compounds that may help reduce inflammation and enhance gut health, linked to mood regulation.

3. Healthy Fats

- **Olive Oil**: Extra virgin olive oil is high in oleocanthal, which has anti-inflammatory effects and supports brain health, contributing to emotional resilience.

- **Avocados**: Packed with healthy fats, fiber, and antioxidants that can promote heart health and enhance mood stability.
- **Nuts** (e.g., walnuts, Brazil nuts, almonds): Rich in omega-3 fatty acids and antioxidants that support brain health and may alleviate symptoms of depression and anxiety.
- **Chia Seeds**: High in omega-3 fatty acids and fiber, promoting heart health and emotional balance.
- **Flaxseeds**: A source of omega-3s and lignans, which may help stabilize mood and reduce inflammation.

4. Spices and Herbs

- **Turmeric**: Contains curcumin, a powerful anti-inflammatory compound that may improve mood and reduce symptoms of anxiety and depression.
- **Ginger**: Known for its anti-inflammatory properties and can help alleviate stress-related digestive issues.
- **Garlic**: Contains sulfur compounds that help reduce inflammation and can enhance the immune system, supporting overall health.
- **Cinnamon**: Known for its anti-inflammatory properties and may help regulate blood sugar levels, which can stabilize mood.
- **Black Pepper**: Enhances the absorption of curcumin from turmeric, amplifying its benefits for mood and emotional health.

5. Whole Proteins

- **Fatty Fish** (e.g., salmon, mackerel, sardines): High in omega-3 fatty acids, which have been shown to reduce symptoms of anxiety and depression.
- **Lean Poultry** (e.g., chicken, turkey): Good sources of protein that support neurotransmitter production, crucial for regulating mood.

- **Legumes** (e.g., lentils, chickpeas, black beans): Rich in fiber and protein that promote gut health, which is linked to improved mental well-being.
- **Eggs**: A great source of protein and nutrients, including vitamin D, which can improve mood and cognitive function.

6. Fermented Foods

Prebiotics and Probiotics: A Quick Overview

Prebiotics are non-digestible fibers that act as food for beneficial gut bacteria, nourishing probiotics and promoting a balanced microbiome essential for digestion and immune health.

Probiotics are live microorganisms that provide health benefits by restoring gut bacteria balance. They improve digestion, enhance immunity, and support mental well-being.

Together, prebiotics and probiotics work synergistically to promote gut health and overall wellness, making them vital for your emotional and physical health.

Garlic: A fantastic prebiotic, garlic feeds the good bacteria in your gut, promoting a healthy microbiome.

Onions: Another great prebiotic, onions help boost gut health by nourishing beneficial gut bacteria.

Asparagus: This vegetable is rich in prebiotic fiber, making it an excellent choice for supporting gut health.

Bananas: A convenient snack, bananas also contain prebiotic fiber that feeds good gut bacteria.

Yogurt: Creamy and delicious, yogurt supports gut health and has been linked to improved mood and reduced anxiety.

Sauerkraut: Fermented cabbage packed with beneficial bacteria, sauerkraut may help stabilize mood and promote emotional resilience.

Kimchi: A spicy fermented dish full of antioxidants, kimchi supports gut health and helps regulate mood.

Kefir: This tangy fermented drink is rich in beneficial microorganisms that support gut health and enhance emotional well-being.

Miso: A flavorful fermented paste made from soybeans, miso is great for gut health and adds depth to soups and dressings.

Tempeh: This fermented soy product is high in protein and probiotics, making it a wonderful addition to meals that promotes gut health.

Pickles: Naturally fermented pickles can be a tasty source of beneficial bacteria that support digestion and mood.

7. Beverages

- **Green Tea:** Contains polyphenols and antioxidants, particularly EGCG, which have calming effects and can help reduce stress.
- **Herbal Teas** (e.g., ginger, chamomile): Can help soothe inflammation and promote relaxation, making them ideal for winding down after a stressful day.
- **Beet Juice:** Known for its high nitrate content, which can help improve circulation and may have a positive impact on mood.

Each of these tools offers unique benefits and can be a valuable part of your healing journey. Explore to find what resonates with you and integrate them into your daily life. Remember, healing is a personal journey and finding the right combination of practices can help you move toward your true, authentic self, far greater than you can imagine.

CONCLUSION

A Heartfelt Thank You

You did it! And I want to extend my deepest gratitude to you. Thank you for taking the time to read this book and for bravely stepping toward your own healing. By engaging with these pages you've embraced vulnerability, self-awareness, and self-compassion, essential elements on the path to growth and transformation.

I commend you for every effort you've made. Each moment of reflection and introspection is a testament to your strength and resilience. Healing is a deeply personal journey and your commitment to it shows your readiness to embrace the fullness of who you are meant to be.

If this book has touched your heart, provided comfort, offered insight—or if it made you smile—I'd love to hear about it. Your feedback means the world to me and can be incredibly helpful to others who might benefit from this journey as well. If you feel inspired to share your thoughts, a review on Amazon can help others discover this book and begin their own journey to healing. Your experience could be just what someone else needs to take the first step.

Remember, this is just the beginning. The insights and tools you've gained are now part of your life, ready to support you as you continue to grow and heal.

You are never alone—there's a community, including mine, cheering you on every step of the way.

Thank you, from the bottom of my heart, for allowing me to be instrumental in your journey. I wish you endless love, peace, and empowerment as you move forward on the path to healing.

With all my love,
Farrah

Dear Former Self,

I see you there, carrying the weight of all that pain, confusion, and longing. You've tried so hard to hold it all together, haven't you? To be strong when the world felt so heavy, to smile when your heart was breaking, and to keep moving forward when all you wanted was to curl up and hide from it all. You've been so brave, so resilient, and yet I know how tired you are— deeply, utterly exhausted.

I want you to know that it's okay to feel everything you've been holding back. It's okay to admit that you're hurting, to acknowledge the fear and sadness that have been buried deep within. You don't have to pretend anymore. You don't have to be the perfect, unshakable version of you that you thought you needed to be because that's what others expected of you. It's okay to let those walls come down, even if just for a moment.

I'm here now, with open arms, ready to hold you in all your messiness, all your beautiful, flawed humanity. You don't need to hide from me because I see you—all of you. I see the little girl who just wanted to feel safe, the young woman who felt lost and alone, the mother who carries the weight of her past while trying to give her children the love she never fully received.

I'm not here to judge you. I'm not here to tell you what you should have done or who you should have been. I'm here to love you, exactly as you are. I'm here to tell you that you are enough, even in your brokenness. You are worthy of love, not despite your pain but because of it. Your scars tell a story of survival, of strength, of a heart that refused to give up, even when it was completely shattered.

It's time to lay down that burden, my dear. It's time to forgive yourself for all the ways you think you've failed, all the times you think you should have been better, stronger, more. You did the best you could with what you had and that is more than enough. You are more than enough.

As you move forward I want you to carry this truth in your heart: You are deserving of peace, of joy, of a life that feels good to live. You don't have to keep reliving the past; don't have to keep punishing yourself for what you couldn't control. You are free to let go, to heal, and to step into the fullness of who you are meant to be.

I love you. I am so proud of you. And I will always, always be here for you.

With all my heart,

_____

(Sign your name)

References

Chapter 1: To Understand Your 'SELF', Start Here

Schwartz, R. C. (1995). Internal family systems therapy. Guilford Press.

Bandler, R., & Grinder, J. (1975). The structure of magic: A book about language and therapy (Vol. 1). Science and Behavior Books.

Chapter 2: The Invisible Load of Motherhood

Ciciolla, L., & Luthar, S. S. (2019). Invisible household labor and ramifications for adjustment: Mothers as captains of households. Sex Roles, 81(7–8), 467–486. https://doi.org/10.1007/s11199-018-1001-x

American Psychological Association. (2022, October 31). How stress affects your health. https://www.apa.org/topics/stress/health

Berman, H., Mason, R., Hall, J., Rodger, S., Classen, C. C., Evans, M. K., Ross, L. E., Mulcahy, G. A., Carranza, L., & Al-Zoubi, F. (2014). Laboring to mother in the context of past trauma. Qualitative Health Research, 24(9), 1253–1264. https://doi.org/10.1177/1049732314521902

Huth-Bocks, A. C., Krause, K., Ahlfs-Dunn, S., Gallagher, E., & Scott, S. (2013). Relational trauma and posttraumatic stress symptoms among pregnant women. Psychodynamic Psychiatry, 41(2), 277–301. https://doi.org/10.1521/pdps.2013.41.2.277

Danese, A., & Lewis, S. J. (2016). Psychoneuroimmunology of early-life stress: The hidden wounds of childhood trauma?

Neuropsychopharmacology, 42(1), 99–114. https://doi.org/10.1038/npp.2016.198

Kugler, B. B., Bloom, M., Kaercher, L. B., Truax, T. V., & Storch, E. A. (2012). Somatic symptoms in traumatized children and adolescents. Child Psychiatry & Human Development, 43(5), 661–673. https://doi.org/10.1007/s10578-012-0289-y

Newhall, C., Hendley II, J. W., & Stauffer, P. H. (1997). The cataclysmic 1991 eruption of Mount Pinatubo, Philippines (U.S. Geological Survey Fact Sheet 113-97). U.S. Department of the Interior, U.S. Geological Survey. https://pubs.usgs.gov/fs/1997/fs113-97/

Chapter 3: The Baggage I Didn't Know I Had

McLeod, S. (2024). Maslow's hierarchy of needs. ResearchGate. https://www.researchgate.net/publication/383241976_Maslow's_Hierarchy_of_Needs

World Health Organization. (n.d.). Coronavirus disease (COVID-19) pandemic in the WHO European region. World Health Organization. https://www.who.int/europe/emergencies/situations/covid-19

Sirois, F. M. (2023). Procrastination and stress: A conceptual review of why context matters. International Journal of Environmental Research and Public Health, 20(6), 5031. https://doi.org/10.3390/ijerph20065031

Tedeschi, R. G., & Calhoun, L. G. (2004). Posttraumatic growth: Conceptual foundations and empirical evidence. Psychological Inquiry, 15(1), 1–18. https://doi.org/10.1207/s15327965pli1501_01

Shapiro, F. (2017). Eye movement desensitization and reprocessing (EMDR) therapy: Basic principles, protocols, and procedures (3rd ed.). Guilford Press.

Viktor Frankl. (n.d.). Viktor Frankl biography.
https://viktorfranklamerica.com/viktor-frankl-bio/

Substance Abuse and Mental Health Services Administration (SAMHSA). (2014). Trauma-informed care in behavioral health services: A review of the literature (Treatment Improvement Protocol [TIP] Series 57). Substance Abuse and Mental Health Services Administration.
https://www.ncbi.nlm.nih.gov/books/NBK207192/

Moffitt, T. E., Arseneault, L., Belsky, D., Dickson, N., Hancox, R. J., Harrington, H., ... & Caspi, A. (2011). A gradient of childhood self-control predicts health, wealth, and public safety. Proceedings of the National Academy of Sciences, 108(7), 2693-2698.
https://doi.org/10.1073/pnas.1010076108

Goleman, D. (1995).

Emotional intelligence: Why it can matter more than IQ. Bantam Books.

van der Kolk, B. A. (2014).

The body keeps the score: Brain, mind, and body in the healing of trauma. Penguin Books.

Moreno, A. L., & Kearney, C. A. (2013). Hypervigilance in children: A new perspective on its measurement and implications for treatment. Journal of Anxiety Disorders, 27(2), 122-129.
https://doi.org/10.1016/j.janxdis.2013.03.005

Lange, B. C. L., Callinan, L. S., & Smith, M. V. (2019). Adverse childhood experiences and their relation to parenting stress and parenting practices. Community Mental Health Journal, 55(4), 651–662. https://doi.org/10.1007/s10597-018-0331-z

Kira, I. A., Lewandowski, L., & Alhassan, A. (2016). Intergenerational trauma: Conceptualization and its relevance to mental health. American Journal of Orthopsychiatry, 86(1), 75–85. https://doi.org/10.1037/ort0000135

BMC Psychiatry. (2024). Effects of childhood trauma on adult mental health: The mediating role of emotion regulation difficulties. BMC Psychiatry. https://doi.org/10.1186/s12888-024-06019-0

Kaufman, E. A. (2021). The impact of maternal childhood trauma on birth experiences: A qualitative study (Master's thesis, University of Tennessee). TRACE. https://trace.tennessee.edu/cgi/viewcontent.cgi?article=2983&context=utk_chanhonoproj

Pinn, T. M., & Marzouk, D. (2023). Birth trauma and its impact on maternal mental health. In Maternal Mental Health in the Postpartum Period (pp. 53-72). Springer. https://doi.org/10.1007/978-3-031-33639-3_4

Richelle, J., & Alea, N. (2023). Stay positive: The effects of positive affect journaling on emotion when remembering COVID-19. Journal of Creativity in Mental Health, 19(4), 529–541. https://doi.org/10.1080/15401383.2023.2281547

American Academy of Pediatrics. (n.d.). Resources for families: Trauma-informed care. https://www.aap.org/en/patient-care/trauma-informed-care/resources-for-families/

Perciavalle, V., Blandini, M., Fecarotta, P., Buscemi, A., Di Corrado, D., Bertolo, L., Fichera, F., & Coco, M. (2016). The role of deep breathing on stress. Neurological Sciences, 37(6), 865–872. https://doi.org/10.1007/s10072-016-2790-8

Maté, G. (2003). When the body says no: Exploring the stress-disease connection. Wiley.

Chapter 4: The Invisible Saboteurs

National Alliance on Mental Illness (NAMI). (n.d.). Understanding triggers. https://nami.org/Your-Journey/Identity-and-Cultural-Dimensions/Understanding-Triggers

Riachi, E., Holma, J., & Laitila, A. (2022). Psychotherapists' views on triggering factors for psychological disorders. Discover Psychology, 2(1), Article 58. https://doi.org/10.1007/s44202-022-00058-y

Substance Abuse and Mental Health Services Administration. (2014). Understanding the impact of trauma. In Trauma-informed care in behavioral health services (pp. 1–21). https://www.ncbi.nlm.nih.gov/books/NBK207191/

Wenzel, A., & Wenzel, S. (2017). The impact of social support on psychological health: A review of recent research. Annual Review of Psychology, 68(1), 535-562. https://doi.org/10.1146/annurev-psych-010416-044208

Woolley, A. (n.d.). The power of unblending in Internal Family Systems therapy. Psychology Today. https://www.psychologytoday.com/us/blog/the-therapy-session/201911/the-power-unblending-internal-family-systems-therapy

Chapter 5: You're Not Okay

Beesley, K. (2022, July 11). "I'm too busy." This might be a reflection of underlying issues. Psychology Today. https://www.psychologytoday.com/us/blog/psychoanalysis-unplugged/202207/the-internal-chaos-of-chronically-busy-people

Curran, T., & Hill, A. P. (2019). Perfectionism is increasing over time: A meta-analysis of birth cohort differences from 1989 to 2016. Psychological Bulletin, 145(4), 410–429. https://doi.org/10.1037/bul0000138

Goldberg, A., & Zibenberg, A. (2024). Parenting an adolescent: The case of the avoidant highly sensitive mother. Child Psychiatry & Human Development. https://doi.org/10.1007/s10578-024-01761-8

Wood, A. M., Froh, J. J., & Geraghty, A. W. (2010). Gratitude and well-being: A review and theoretical integration. Clinical Psychology Review, 30(7), 890-905. https://doi.org/10.1016/j.cpr.2010.03.005

Hay, L. (1984). You can heal your life. Hay House.

Chapter 6: Your Brain Isn't Your Bestie

Emmons, R. A. (2007). Thanks! How the new science of gratitude can make you happier. Houghton Mifflin Harcourt.

Seligman, M. E. P. (2002). Authentic happiness: Using the new positive psychology to realize your potential for lasting fulfillment. Free Press.

Seligman, M. E. P. (2011). Flourish: A visionary new understanding of happiness and well-being. Free Press.

Maltz, M. (1960). Psycho-cybernetics. New York, NY: Prentice Hall.

Cumming, J., & Williams, S. E. (2013). The role of imagery in performance. Journal of Imagery Research in Sport and Physical Activity, 8(1). https://doi.org/10.1515/jirspa-2013-0001

Wang, H., Zhang, S., & Gu, Y. (2021). The role of self-affirmation in alleviating the effects of stress on mental health among adults: A systematic review and meta-analysis. Frontiers in Psychology, 12, 1-12. https://doi.org/10.3389/fpsyg.2021.751803

Harris, P. R., & Napper, L. (2005). Self-affirmation and health behavior: A review of the literature. Health Psychology Review, 1(2), 104-129. https://doi.org/10.1080/17437199.2015.1012345

Cascio, C. N., O'Donnell, M. B., Tinney, F. J., Lieberman, M. D., Taylor, S. E., Strecher, V. J., & Falk, E. B. (2016). Self-affirmation activates brain systems associated with self-related processing and reward and is reinforced by future orientation. Social Cognitive and Affective Neuroscience, 11(4), 621–629. https://doi.org/10.1093/scan/nsv136

Dutcher, J. M., Creswell, J. D., Pacilio, L. E., Harris, P. R., Klein, W. M. P., Levine, J. M., Bower, J. E., Muscatell, K. A., & Eisenberger, N. I. (2016). Self-affirmation activates the ventral striatum. Psychological Science, 27(4), 455–466. https://doi.org/10.1177/0956797615625989

Yu, J., Yang, Z., Sun, S., Sun, K., Chen, W., Zhang, L., Xu, J., Xu, Q., Liu, Z., Ke, J., Zhang, L., & Zhu, Y. (2024). The effect of weighted blankets on sleep and related disorders: a brief review. Frontiers in psychiatry, 15, 1333015. https://doi.org/10.3389/fpsyt.2024.1333015

Daukantaitė, D., Tellhed, U., Maddux, R. E., Svensson, T., & Melander, O. (2018). Five-week yin yoga-based interventions decreased plasma adrenomedullin and increased psychological health in stressed adults: A randomized controlled trial. PLOS ONE, 13(7), Article e0200518. https://doi.org/10.1371/journal.pone.0200518

Tam, C. S., Johnson, W. D., Rood, J., Heaton, A. L., & Greenway, F. L. (2020). Increased human growth hormone after oral consumption of an amino acid supplement: Results of a randomized, placebo-controlled, double-blind, crossover study in healthy subjects. American Journal of Therapeutics, 27(4), e333–e337. https://doi.org/10.1097/MJT.0000000000000893

Hale, L., & Guan, S. (2015). Screen time and sleep among school-aged children and adolescents: A systematic literature review. Sleep Medicine Reviews, 21, 50–58. https://doi.org/10.1016/j.smrv.2014.07.007

Hill, N. (1937). Think and grow rich. The Ralston Society.

Chapter 7: Life Happens for You

Seligman, M. E. P. (2006). Learned optimism: How to change your mind and your life. Vintage.

Learning about thought reframing. (n.d.). My Health Alberta. https://myhealth.alberta.ca/Health/aftercareinformation/pages/conditions.aspx?hwid=abk7438

Allison, P. J., Guichard, C., Fung, K., & Gilain, L. (2003). Dispositional optimism predicts survival status 1 year after diagnosis in head and neck cancer patients. Journal of Clinical Oncology, 21(3), 543–548. https://doi.org/10.1200/JCO.2003.10.092

Segerstrom, S. C., & Sephton, S. E. (2010). Optimistic expectancies and cell-mediated immunity. Psychological Science, 21(3), 448–455. https://doi.org/10.1177/0956797610362061

Cleveland Clinic. (2022, September 19). What is negative self-talk and how to change it. https://health.clevelandclinic.org/what-is-negative-self-talk-and-how-to-change-it

Shaw, K. D., Manzella, F., & McCarthy, D. M. (2021). Enhancing emotion regulation through exposure therapy: The role of memory specificity and cognitive reappraisal in youth with anxiety. Frontiers in Psychology, 12, Article 706037. https://doi.org/10.3389/fpsyg.2021.706037

Chapter 8: Self-Care Unplugged: Am I Being True to Myself?

Sutton, R. I. (2018, January 9). What self-awareness really is and how to cultivate it. Harvard Business Review. https://hbr.org/2018/01/what-self-awareness-really-is-and-how-to-cultivate-it

Carden, J., Jones, R. J., & Passmore, J. (2021). Defining self-awareness in the context of adult development: A systematic literature review. Organizational Behavior Teaching Review, 46(1), 140–177. https://doi.org/10.1177/1052562921990065

Anderson, D. E., Kuehn, J. L., & Matz, J. (2021). An overview of the use of the self-awareness and self-reflection in nursing practice: Implications for nurse education. Nurse Education in Practice, 52, 103018. https://doi.org/10.1016/j.nepr.2021.103018

Harris, M. A., & Casey, M. M. (2021). A reflective inquiry into self-awareness and the importance of mindfulness in higher education. The Journal of Teaching and Learning, 15(1), 47–58. https://doi.org/10.5325/jteachlearn.15.1.0047

Ranabir, S., & Reetu, K. (2011). Stress and hormones. Indian Journal of Endocrinology and Metabolism, 15(1), 18–22. https://doi.org/10.4103/2230-8210.77573

Gupta, M. A. (2013). Review of somatic symptoms in post-traumatic stress disorder. International Review of Psychiatry, 25(1), 86–99. https://doi.org/10.3109/09540261.2012.736367

Kugler, B.B., Bloom, M., Kaercher, L.B. et al. Somatic Symptoms in Traumatized Children and Adolescents. Child Psychiatry Hum Dev 43, 661–673 (2012). https://doi.org/10.1007/s10578-012-0289-y

Brown, B. (2015). Daring greatly: How the courage to be vulnerable transforms the way we live, love, parent, and lead (Paperback ed.). Gotham Books.

Chapter 9: Calm Blueprint

Covey, S. R. (1989). The 7 habits of highly effective people: Powerful lessons in personal change. Free Press.

Dhabhar, F. S. (2014). Effects of stress on immune function: The good, the bad, and the beautiful. Immunology Research, 58(2), 193–210. https://doi.org/10.1007/s12026-014-8517-0

Ganapathi, P., Aithal, S., & Kanchana, D. (2023). Stress management: Concept, approaches, and analysis. International Journal of Management, Technology, and Social Sciences, 213-222. https://doi.org/10.47992/IJMTS.2581.6012.0319

I'm So Stressed Out! Fact Sheet. (n.d.). National Institute of Mental Health (NIMH). https://www.nimh.nih.gov/health/publications/so-stressed-out-fact-sheet

Hubbs, D. L., & Brand, C. F. (2005). The paper mirror: Understanding reflective journaling. Journal of Experiential Education, 28(1), 60–71. https://doi.org/10.1177/105382590502800107

Smyth, J. M., Johnson, J. A., Auer, B. J., Lehman, E., Talamo, G., & Sciamanna, C. N. (2018). Online positive affect journaling in the improvement of mental distress and well-being in general medical patients with elevated anxiety symptoms: A preliminary randomized controlled trial. JMIR Mental Health, 5(4), e11290. https://doi.org/10.2196/11290

Chapter 10: Creating a Supportive Environment

Moore, S. (Host). (2023). Let it be easy with Susie Moore [Audio podcast episode]. In Let it be easy. Apple Podcasts. https://podcasts.apple.com/us/podcast/let-it-be-easy-with-susie-moore/id1614486542

Treatment, C. F. S. A. (2014). Trauma-informed care: A sociocultural perspective. In Trauma-informed care in behavioral health services (pp. 1-11). NCBI Bookshelf. https://www.ncbi.nlm.nih.gov/books/NBK207195/

Maraz, A., Griffiths, M. D., & Demetrovics, Z. (2016). The prevalence of compulsive buying: A meta-analysis. Addiction, 111(3), 408–419. https://doi.org/10.1111/add.13223

Lejoyeux, M., Tassain, V., Solomon, J., & Adès, J. (1997). Study of compulsive buying in depressed patients. The Journal of Clinical Psychiatry, 58(4), 169–173. https://doi.org/10.4088/jcp.v58n0406

Zhao, J., Jia, T., Wang, X., Xiao, Y., & Wu, X. (2022). Risk factors associated with social media addiction: An exploratory study. Frontiers in Psychology, 13, 837766. https://doi.org/10.3389/fpsyg.2022.837766

Chapter 11: Setting Boundaries with Love

Lanius, R. A., Terpou, B. A., & McKinnon, M. C. (2020). The sense of self in the aftermath of trauma: Lessons from the default mode network in posttraumatic stress disorder. European Journal of Psychotraumatology, 11(1), 1807703. https://doi.org/10.1080/20008198.2020.1807703

EndCAN. (2023, October 23). The importance of setting boundaries as an adult survivor of child abuse. EndCAN. https://endcan.org/2023/10/23/the-importance-of-setting-boundaries-as-an-adult-survivor-of-child-abuse/

Cloud, H., & Townsend, J. (2017). Boundaries: Updated and expanded edition: When to say yes, how to say no to take control of your life. Zondervan.

National Center for Complementary and Integrative Health (NCCIH). (2024). Mind and body approaches for stress and anxiety: What the science says. https://www.nccih.nih.gov

Wilson-Mendenhall, C. D., & Dunne, J. D. (2021). Cultivating emotional granularity. Frontiers in Psychology, 12. https://doi.org/10.3389/fpsyg.2021.703658

Goleman, D. (1995). Emotional intelligence: Why it can matter more than IQ. Bantam Books.

Koch, S. C., & Fisher, A. (2018). Embodiment and trauma: A relational and neurological perspective. Frontiers in Neuroscience, 12, Article 70. https://doi.org/10.3389/fnins.2018.00070

Joseph, B., Wynne, J. L., Dudrick, S. J., & Hurst, S. (2010). Nutrition in trauma and critically ill patients. European Journal of Trauma, 36(1), 25–30. https://doi.org/10.1007/s00068-010-9213-y

Bullmore, E. (2018). The inflamed mind: A radical new approach to depression. Picador.

Du, J., Zhu, M., Bao, H., Li, B., Dong, Y., Xiao, C., Zhang, G. Y., Henter, I., Rudorfer, M., & Vitiello, B. (2016). The role of nutrients in protecting mitochondrial function and neurotransmitter signaling: Implications for the treatment of depression, PTSD, and suicidal behaviors. Critical Reviews in Food Science and Nutrition, 56(15), 2560–2578. https://doi.org/10.1080/10408398.2013.876960

Chapter 12: Embracing and Transforming Shame, Guilt, and Anger

Torstveit, L., Sütterlin, S., & Lugo, R. G. (2016). Empathy, guilt proneness, and gender: Relative contributions to prosocial behavior. Europe's Journal of Psychology, 12(2), 260–270. https://doi.org/10.5964/ejop.v12i2.1097

López-Castro, T., Saraiya, T., Zumberg-Smith, K., & Dambreville, N. (2019). Association between shame and posttraumatic stress disorder: A meta-analysis. Journal of Traumatic Stress, 32(4), 484–495. https://doi.org/10.1002/jts.22411

DeCou, C. R., Lynch, S. M., Weber, S., Richner, D., Mozafari, A., Huggins, H., & Perschon, B. (2023). On the association between trauma-related shame and symptoms of psychopathology: A meta-analysis. Trauma, Violence, & Abuse, 24(3), 1193–1201. https://doi.org/10.1177/15248380211053617

Brown, B. (2012). Daring Greatly: How the Courage to Be Vulnerable Transforms the Way We Live, Love, Parent, and Lead. Gotham Books.

Neff, K. (2011). Self-Compassion: The Proven Power of Being Kind to Yourself. William Morrow.

Tangney, J. P., & Dearing, R. L. (2002). Emotion, Shame, and Guilt. Guilford Press.

Stotz, S. J., Elbert, T., Müller, V., & Schauer, M. (2015). The relationship between trauma, shame, and guilt: Findings from a community-based study of refugee minors in Germany. European Journal of Psychotraumatology, 6(1). https://doi.org/10.3402/ejpt.v6.25863

Bradshaw, J. (2005). Healing the shame that binds you. HarperCollins.

Wolynn, M. (2016). It didn't start with you: How inherited family trauma shapes who we are and how to end the cycle. Penguin Press.

Win, E., Zainal, N. H., & Newman, M. G. (2021). Trait anger expression mediates childhood trauma predicting adulthood anxiety, depressive, and alcohol use disorders. Journal of Affective Disorders, 288, 114–121. https://doi.org/10.1016/j.jad.2021.03.086

Chapter 13: Embracing Self-Compassion

Scheffers, M., Hoek, M., Bosscher, R. J., van Duijn, M. A. J., Schoevers, R. A., & van Busschbach, J. T. (2017). Negative body experience in women with early childhood trauma: Associations with trauma severity and dissociation. European Journal of Psychotraumatology, 8(1). https://doi.org/10.1080/20008198.2017.1322892

Malecki, J., Rhodes, P., & Ussher, J. (2018). Childhood trauma and anorexia nervosa: From body image to embodiment. Health Care for Women International, 39(8), 936–951. https://doi.org/10.1080/07399332.2018.1492268

Lawn, R. B., Murchland, A. R., Kim, Y., Chibnik, L. B., Tworoger, S. S., Rimm, E. B., Sumner, J. A., Roberts, A. L., Nishimi, K. M.,

Ratanatharathorn, A. D., Jha, S. C., Koenen, K. C., & Kubzansky, L. D. (2022). Trauma, psychological distress and markers of systemic inflammation among US women: A longitudinal study. Psychoneuroendocrinology, 145, 105915. https://doi.org/10.1016/j.psyneuen.2022.105915

Aas, M., Ueland, T., Inova, A., Melle, I., Andreassen, O. A., & Steen, N. E. (2020). Childhood trauma is nominally associated with elevated cortisol metabolism in severe mental disorder. Frontiers in Psychiatry, 11, Article 391. https://doi.org/10.3389/fpsyt.2020.00391

Grebenciucova, E., & VanHaerents, S. (2023). Interleukin 6: at the interface of human health and disease. Frontiers in Immunology, 14. https://doi.org/10.3389/fimmu.2023.1255533

Miller, A. H., & Raison, C. L. (2016). The role of inflammation in depression: From evolutionary imperative to modern treatment target. Nature Reviews Immunology, 16(1), 22–34. https://doi.org/10.1038/nri.2015.5

Adam, T. C., & Epel, E. S. (2007). Stress, eating, and the reward system. Physiology & Behavior, 91(4), 449–458. https://doi.org/10.1016/j.physbeh.2007.04.011

Chapter 14: The Weight of Your Own Story

Sjblom, M., ضhrling, K., Prellwitz, M., & Kostenius, C. (2016). Health throughout the lifespan: The phenomenon of the inner child reflected in events during childhood experienced by older persons. International Journal of Qualitative Studies on Health and Well-Being, 11, Article 31486. https://doi.org/10.3402/qhw.v11.31486

Bradshaw, J. (1990). Homecoming: Reclaiming and championing your inner child. HarperCollins.

Avis, K. A., Stroebe, M., & Schut, H. (2021). Stages of grief portrayed on the internet: A systematic analysis and critical appraisal. Frontiers in Psychology, 12, Article 772696. https://doi.org/10.3389/fpsyg.2021.772696

Kanji, S., & Cahusac, E. (2015). Who am I? Mothers' shifting identities, loss and sensemaking after workplace exit. Human Relations, 68(9), 1415–1436. https://doi.org/10.1177/0018726714557336

Minton, E. A., Wang, C. X., Anthony, C. M., & Fox, A. K. (2023). The process model of stigmatized loss: Identity-threatened experiences of bereaved mothers. Qualitative Health Research, 33(14), 1262–1278. https://doi.org/10.1177/10497323231203643

Kim, J. J., Payne, E. S., & Tracy, E. L. (2022). Indirect effects of forgiveness on psychological health through anger and hope: A parallel mediation analysis. Journal of Religion and Health, 61(5), 3729–3746. https://doi.org/10.1007/s10943-022-01518-4

Acknowledgements

To my beloved husband and my children.
I dedicate this success to each of you.
I love you all with all my heart.

My parents.
Thank you for bringing me to this world.
My siblings.
Your presence in my life has influenced the person I am today.
And for that, I am grateful.
My in-laws.
Your kindness and love have enriched my life in ways
I will forever cherish.

To those who have walked beside me,
Past, present and future,
Thank you for leaving your mark on my story.

My Heavenly Father.
Your love is unwavering, your guidance and grace is infinite.
Thank you for the courage and strength when I couldn't go on.
For the blessings and wisdom you continue to bestow on me.
To you belong all the glory.

The unfolding of "*Baggage: Claimed*" - Chapter one (Unedited)

Suddenly, chaos erupts. A drink crashes to the floor, sending ice and liquid splattering across nearby chairs and mercilessly staining someone's pristine Louboutins. The sound cuts through the ambient buzz of chatter, drawing startled glances from onlookers, but for a moment, it feels like no one blinks—as if time itself has stuttered before catching up. Their wide eyes reflect disbelief, caught in the unexpected moment.

Apologies spill forth like the drink, frantic and overlapping, but the damage is irreversible. Those red soles, once symbols of elegance, are now marred—a stark reminder of how swiftly fortune can turn. The air feels charged, a mix of shock and the lingering scent of spilled soda, as everyone momentarily holds their breath.

"I'm so, so sorry!" I blurt out, my face flushing hot with embarrassment. My voice sounds faint to my ears, almost as if it's coming from far away, distant and detached. **What a disaster!** I think to myself, wishing I could just disappear. Suddenly, a flash—I'm not at the café anymore. I'm on the plane. No, wait. I'm back here. That woman is still glaring at me.

"Honestly, do you have any idea how much these cost?" the woman retorts, her voice dripping with condescension. **Well, if they were on sale...** I quip silently, trying to mask my rising anxiety as she looks me up and down, her disdain palpable.

"I really didn't see you," I reply, my heart racing. "Please let me make it up to you!"

"Make it up to me?" she scoffs. **What does she expect me to do?**

As her words hang in the air, a flush of humiliation sweeps over me. The buzzing sound in the café grows louder, oppressive. Is it always this loud? Or is it just in my head? I take a deep cleansing breath, forcing myself to look away from her scornful gaze. The café buzzes around us, life resuming in a blur of fragmented conversations and the clatter of ceramic cups against saucers.

The aroma of roasted beans mingles with stale perfume that lingers like a half-hearted compliment. But now the perfume smells wrong, too sharp, too metallic. It claws at the back of my throat. It's a heady concoction that barely disguises the faint whiff of jet fuel wafting in from the terminal doors. Soft bossa nova floats from the speakers, trying to convince us we're lounging in a trendy Brazilian café rather than marooned in an airport. As if that smooth rhythm could make us feel chic while we're really just disheveled and confused.

The fluorescent lights above flutter intermittently, flickering too rapidly now, casting sharp reflections off the polished floor like flashes of broken memories. The lights pulse to the beat of my heart, or maybe it's the other way around. The floor beneath my feet seems to dip slightly, as if the ground is not as solid as it should be. I grip my chair. **Am I moving?** Everything feels just a bit too bright, too polished, like a too-enthusiastic host trying to make small talk at a party where nobody knows each other. Except here, I'm not sure I know myself either. This place is trying so hard to be more than it is—just like me, desperately clinging to clarity while the world around me spins in dizzying circles.

My flight is delayed, and as I sip my sparkling water, the bubbles seem to explode louder than normal—fizzing against my lips as if trying to break free. I can't help but roll my eyes at the irony. I used to enjoy caramel macchiatos with extra foam, but today I seek clarity. The last thing I want when flying is dehydration, both of body and spirit.

Okay, deep breaths. Breathe in, breathe out. It's just an airport, not a pressure cooker. I remind myself, feeling my nervous system slowly settle now that the Louboutin lady has vanished. But even with her gone, the prickling sensation on the back of my neck lingers. *Are they still looking at me? Do they think I'm a total klutz?* I can almost hear the whispers of judgment floating around, swirling like the ambient noise of the café.

Glancing around, I take in the eclectic mix of travelers, each with their own story of delay and disappointment. A young couple clutches their boarding passes, eyes fixed on the screens, hoping for a miracle. An older man, slumped in his chair, exudes a sense of resignation; his flight had already been delayed for hours.

Maybe they think I'm some kind of circus act, too clumsy to belong here.

We're all just pawns in the game of air travel, subject to the whims of the airlines and the weather. My own story is just one of many, a small thread in the complex accouterment of travelers stuck in this endless cycle of waiting.

This is LAX, after all—the city of angels, where dreams are delayed as often as flights. Between the palm trees and plastic smiles, it's all too easy to get swept up in the mirage. It's like Hollywood on layover, where reality is a prop and everyone is auditioning for a role they believe they've already secured. *But what role am I playing? I catch my reflection in the café's glass wall, and for a split second, I don't recognize the person staring back.*

I watch the parade of hopefuls and has-beens shuffle past, wheeling their designer luggage like it's a badge of honor. Their faces blur and fade as they pass, expressions indistinct, their motions too smooth, like figures on a moving conveyor belt. A woman in oversized sunglasses and yoga pants scrolls furiously through her phone, her sun-kissed skin and tense jawline suggesting she's balancing both a juice cleanse and an existential crisis.

In this hub of dreams and illusions, I'm captivated by the diverse cast of characters surrounding me. There's a man nearby with a cravat tied just so, ankle pants that flirt with the line of fashion-forward, and sockless loafers that scream confidence. If confidence had a scent, it would be citrus and sandalwood, something like Tom Ford. I don't need to be near him to catch a whiff; I know it well because I just spent an hour inhaling every perfume and cologne at Duty Free. He looks like money, smells like money, and swirls his untouched espresso as if it's a prop in his own elaborate performance.

His fingers drum lightly against the porcelain, a subtle rhythm of impatience that betrays the stillness in his posture. **What's he waiting for? Or just a good reason to ignore the rest of us plebeians?** Every so often, his gaze flickers to the departures board, searching for something that isn't there. Behind him, a girl with neon-dyed hair styled like a vibrant explosion clutches a well-worn script, her ripped jeans fraying at the edges as if they reflect her own fraying hopes. *I wonder if she knows her script is more put together than I am right now. I'd probably just mess up my lines.* She mouths her lines, lost in a world of "what ifs," while he sits in his cocoon of privilege, oblivious to the weight of her unfulfilled dreams.

It strikes me that while he has the world at his feet—his expensive loafers sparkling like status symbols—she's left to chase shadows, rehearsing for an audience that may never arrive. In a city where success is often measured by wealth, it's a stark reminder of the deep divide: one person drowning in luxury while the other clings desperately to the fragile hope of a breakthrough. It's a heartbreaking tableau, revealing how the pursuit of dreams can feel like a lottery, where some are born winners and others are left to navigate the weight of unfulfilled aspirations, grappling with setbacks that seem insurmountable. The journey is characterized by quiet struggles, unseen battles, and the relentless search for validation in a world that frequently ignores them.

Outside, planes roar overhead, whisking people away to places they've only seen on Instagram, while others, like me, remain stuck in limbo. It's as if the very essence of LA has seeped into this terminal—a place where people come to escape or be discovered, only to find themselves waiting endlessly. But now the terminal feels endless, too—the walls stretching, the doors multiplying. How long have I been here?

I glance at my watch and think, isn't that just so LA? Always on the cusp of something, but never quite arriving.

Nearby, a child twirls with arms flung wide, laughter cutting through the airport din like birdsong at dawn. Each spin seems to erase another second of time, making me momentarily envious of his carefree joy. He has no past weighing him down, no invisible strings pulling him in ten different directions. Just the joy of the moment, his loose shirt flaring out like a cape, making him feel invincible in a space filled with uncertainty. It's a reminder of what it means to be free—at least until the next announcement breaks the spell.

Here, everyone's chasing something—fame, fortune, or maybe just the perfect vegan latte. But soon, I'll board a flight to a destination that feels more like a necessary obligation than an exciting adventure. If I can find the right gate. Or the right terminal. The signs seem to change every time I look at them, flickering from one destination to the next.

The shadows linger, stretching further than I'd like to admit, and what should be a moment of anticipation is overshadowed by a quiet uncertainty. It's not just the unknown that unsettles me; it's something deeper. The excitement I'd expect to feel is muted, buried beneath an ache I thought I had left behind.

As I sit there, lost in my thoughts, a gentle tap on my shoulder startles me back to reality. I turn to see an elderly woman, her silver hair neatly coiffed, a kind smile crinkling the corners of her eyes.

"Excuse me, dear," she says softly, ***"but I couldn't help noticing you seem a bit troubled. Is everything alright?"*** Her voice echoes slightly, though she's standing right in front of me.

For a moment, I'm taken aback by her concern. In this sea of strangers, each wrapped up in their own dramas, her genuine interest feels like a lifeline. I hesitate, unsure whether to burden this sweet lady with my problems.

"Oh, it's nothing," I begin, but the words feel hollow even as they leave my lips. ***"Just... airport stress, I suppose."***

She nods knowingly, settling into the seat beside me. ***"Ah, yes. These places have a way of... stirring up all sorts of emotions, don't they?"***

She pauses, her gaze drifting to the boy still spinning nearby. ***"But they can also be a place of new beginnings."***

I find myself nodding, surprisingly comforted by her presence. The air around her feels different, heavy like it's charged with static, yet somehow soothing, too.***"It's just... I'm heading somewhere I'm not sure I want to go,"*** I admit, the words tumbling out before I can stop them. I follow her gaze, watching the child's carefree dance. ***"I suppose you're right,"*** I admit, feeling a small smile tug at the corners of my mouth and a sigh heavier than my carry-on.

The woman's eyes soften. Her expression is too kind, too patient, as if she's seen this exact scene play out before.***"Sometimes the journeys we dread the most are the ones that shape us the most,"*** she says, patting my hand gently.

"I remember when I was about your age, I had to fly across the country for my father's funeral. I was terrified of facing the grief, the family tensions, all of it. Oh, my dear. Going home can be the hardest journey of all. We think we've moved on, grown beyond our roots, but those old feelings have a way of sneaking up on us". Her voice feels oddly rehearsed, like lines from a play she's performed a thousand times. I wonder if she even exists outside this moment, outside this airport.

"You know," she continues, her voice warm and rich with experience, *"I've been coming to this airport for over fifty years. Seen all sorts of people, all kinds of stories. And let me tell you, dear, everyone here is carrying something."*

Her words resonate, striking a chord deep within me. I turn to face her fully, suddenly eager to hear more.

She leans in conspiratorially. *"See that businessman over there? The one with the crisp suit and shiny shoes?"* I nod, knowing too well who she's referring to.

"Well," she continues, her eyes twinkling, *"I've seen him here before. Every few months, like clockwork. Always with that same briefcase, always looking so important. But do you know what I noticed?"*

I shake my head, intrigued. But more than that—I'm compelled. There's something in her voice that hooks me, keeps me tethered to her every word.

"He always stops at that little gift shop over there," she points discreetly, *"and buys the same thing. A small, plush teddy bear. Now, why do you think a man like that would need so many stuffed animals?"*

I ponder this for a moment, my own troubles momentarily forgotten. *"Maybe...*

Manufactured by Amazon.ca
Acheson, AB